APPLE CIDER VINEGAR:
A Modern Folk Remedy

APPLE CIDER VINEGAR:
A Modern Folk Remedy

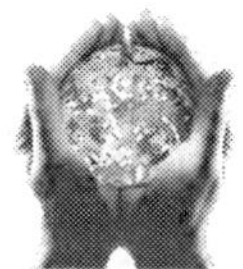

An Earth Clinic Publication

Deirdre Layne, Founder Earth Clinic
Daniel P. Kray
for **Body Axis, LLC**

Body Axis, LLC.
Atlanta

Library of Congress Control Number: 2010934686

Cover design by Christina Rahr Lane
Book design by Denise Wellenstein

DISCLAIMER
The preparation and publication of this book has been undertaken with great care. However, the book is offered for informational purposes only and cannot be taken as a substitute for professional medical prevention, diagnosis, or treatment. Please consult with your physician, pharmacist, or health care provider before taking any home remedies or supplements or following any treatment suggested by anyone within this book. Only your health care provider, personal physician, or pharmacist can provide you with advice on what is safe and effective for your unique needs or diagnose your particular medical history.

Reader feedback taken from the EarthClinic.com website and included in this book is the opinion of the reader alone and does not necessarily reflect the opinions or beliefs of Body Axis LLC, Earth Clinic LLC, this book, or its authors.

Visit us online at:
www.bodyaxis.com
www.earthclinic.com

Printed in the United States of America

FIRST PRINTING: 2010

ISBN-978-0-9828963-0-3

CONTENTS

Chapter One

WELCOME TO THE EARTH CLINIC COMMUNITY!

You might be joining Earth Clinic for the first time with this book, or perhaps you have been with us online from the very start. In any case, you are a welcome part of the Earth Clinic Community. EarthClinic.com, an alternative health and healing site, was launched on the web in 1999 as a local site for our founder, Deirdre Layne's healing practice. It only grew into the internet hotspot it has become because people took interest in the idea of simple, effective, tried-and-true remedies and the idea of sharing them with each other. Except that the people of that community contributed their ideas and experiences, the site would never have been more than a few happy, healthy people out there talking in circles about the one little amazing remedy that started it all.

Apple Cider Vinegar was that first remedy.

Deirdre had a healing practice in Los Angeles at the time, supported by a miniscule website advertising her services in the busy whir of California life and business. With her allergies acting up during one particular spin through that maelstrom, Deirdre came across the health benefits of apple cider vinegar, was convinced to try it out against her allergy symptoms, and then posted her experiences on the website simply as an aside. And that was that, the start of an entirely different crazy storm of interest and vibrant energy that has made EarthClinic.com an international Top Five Alternative Health site on the internet. Earth Clinic has since become a community of shared knowledge — generations and nations full of it — that has brought health and hope through safe, inexpensive, natural cures and home remedies to people around the world. All of them have been contributed, tried, and reported on by regular people just like you.

All Well and Good, but Why Should You Trust Us?

Yes, that is as good and fair a question as any, and an important one in the medical and health business — a place where enormous amounts of money can be made with the right drug, treatment, or well-advertised snake oil. Earth Clinic is different, we promise you that, and we think we've proven it through the years. Not only are the members of our community the major contributors of our cures and feedback, but they are also our only constituents. We take no money from any businesses. We don't accept advertising except through disinterested third parties (like Google advertising systems), and what we offer is generally so cheap (even free) that no one could be expected to make a fortune off it. In all honesty, Earth Clinic never started out to become any sort of business of its own or even something we intended to spend much time on. It was chance alone that saw ACV attract so much attention and then so many other reader contributions on alternative health and folk medicine, so that the site took on a life of its own.

Earth Clinic simply blossomed from that first uncertain apple seed into an orchard full of effective, home-tested, and community-vetted remedies and cures proven through years on the site and before that in the homes of commonsense families for centuries. Eventually, so many cures began to accumulate that Earth Clinic became a responsibility, a collection of cures and remedies so good that it was our duty to share them with as many people as we could. That is the reason you hold this book in your hands right now, as the first and probably most important of the remedies we intend to bring to a wider community than even the internet can hold.

We appreciate that community more than we can express, and each day we happily dedicate more time to this growing group of folks because of people like our friend Goji, from London, who wrote to tell us:

> "I've just reached the ripe old age of 72 years, but inwardly still feel 20. However, over the last few months I have been having problems finding enough energy to get through household and other tasks and, well life had lost its magic. I felt like an old person. In the past I'd tried a well-known brand of ACV, but it did nothing to help how I felt. Then about a fortnight ago I came across an iconic brand (I'm not allowed to mention names) of raw, unfiltered ACV containing the Mother, and I began taking one tablespoon in water sweetened with stevia three times a day just before meals. I now wake up with a song in my heart, the world has suddenly become beautiful again, and my energy has been restored. And I feel the way I walk has become more free, looser somehow, as though I am walking more like a younger person."

We believe you can trust Earth Clinic for two principle reasons. First, many of our completely natural cures cost you no more than a buck apiece, so you have little enough to lose. Furthermore, we have no interest in being the one to collect that dollar from you. That's how we're different, not a billion-dollar biotech trying to foist an expensive half-cure off on you.

The second and more important reason is how seriously we take the idea of community. Earth Clinic is nothing more or less than a collection of friends and helpful neighbors who know that we find safety only as we lead each other toward mutual health and happiness. The cures we are bringing to you here are the cures that first were brought to us, the same cures we have used ourselves. We wouldn't steer you wrong, because someday we'll be depending on you to steer us in the right direction in turn.

How Earth Clinic Works

We began as a healing practice, one that was always interested in other and better healing practices, and if you're looking for a world full of time-tested ideas on how to naturally restore and promote your own health and the health of your family, the internet really is the place to start. No other medium for communication makes it so easy to invite in age-old secrets from around the world — whether it's from a Korean apple cider vinegar maker, a Russian proponent for beets, or a woman from New Zealand who can tell you about a curative plant you'd never heard of before. Hand-me-down remedies started to arrive so quickly in succession that the problem became how exactly to tell which were the good ideas out of all those sent in to the site.

When we recently decided to offer the absolute best of all those natural health remedies in this more accessible printed form, that need to sift the grain from the chaff became even more critical. Fortunately, a process has long been in place to help bring the very most dependable and successful remedies to our attention. That process quite simply is to tally how often a particular remedy has worked, for how many people, and in how many different ways it has improved the lives of our readers and contributors in the community.

The Earth Clinic site has always been a democratic one. Once readers contribute an idea for a cure or remedy, we leave it open to our community members to try the remedy themselves, see whether it works for them, and then ask them to report back with their reviews. It has been through the process of evaluating all that feedback that we've put together a system we find clear enough: if readers have gotten good results, they give the remedy a **Yea**, a **Nay** if it didn't work, or a **Maybe** if their health didn't turn out too clearly for the better or the worse after that particular folk medical treatment. Given a little time, the cream of all possible cures tends to rise to the top, but the fact of the matter is that every bit of wisdom and experience is liable to prove beneficial to someone in our community of health.

In our experience, what we find (and what somehow expensive medical science hasn't figured out) is that people differ in what they need and how they react to different remedies. For some, cayenne pepper will be just the thing they were looking for, but it won't do a thing for the guy who simply needed to add a bit of honey to his diet for the same condition. We're all different, inside and out, and that's why Earth Clinic gives you more than one option to pursue for most conditions, and we give you the straight skinny from our readers themselves so that you can find the person whose condition sounds most like your own.

Why Apple Cider Vinegar?

Okay then, if the Earth Clinic site is so bursting with shared wisdom, why present a book on apple cider vinegar alone? Well, after all, the site began with apple cider vinegar. That wasn't a simple bit of chance but the best of all possible luck, kismet, serendipity, or (we can only hope) good karma. Apple Cider Vinegar (ACV is what we most often call it around here) has become the very first option most of our community turns to almost regardless of what health concern presents itself. ACV isn't a cure-all, nothing is, but we haven't found any other thing that does so much for so many people at so little cost in terms of either money or side effects.

Apple Cider Vinegar, among the oldest and most treasured of the world's home remedies, cures more ailments than any other folk remedy – years of international contributions and personal experience have us convinced. That running process of tabulating the Yeas and Nays of personal experience on the website brought ACV head and shoulders above the competition and straight to our attention for more research and the comprehensive presentation of apple cider vinegar as a modern folk remedy, as we will be presenting it in this book.

We've received extensive feedback on all our remedies over the past ten years, but the reported cures from consuming and applying Apple Cider Vinegar are by far the most numerous. They include cures for allergies (including pet, food and environmental), sinus infections, acne, high cholesterol, flu, chronic fatigue, candida, acid reflux, sore throats, contact dermatitis, arthritis, and even gout (who knew that people still come down with gout?).

Many readers enjoy the fact that apple cider vinegar breaks down fats, and so it is widely used to help us lose weight. It also has been reported that a daily dose of apple cider vinegar can bring high blood pressure under control within two weeks! Apple Cider Vinegar is wonderful for pets, including dogs, cats, and horses. It ameliorates their arthritic conditions, controls fleas & barn flies, and gives a beautiful shine to their coats.

Now for certain, this is vinegar and not a spoonful of sugar. Some folks take to the flavor immediately — and in particular children seem naturally to crave it when offered — but even in the small amounts your body needs, frequent doses of apple cider vinegar can be a tough sell. If you can get over your fears about the taste of apple cider vinegar, you will find it one of the most important natural remedies in healing the body. In fact, you would be in a small minority if you weren't soon trying to explain to friends and family about how much you've come to enjoy its flavor. Then again, maybe they'll just see it in your face — as a wonderful side effect of drinking apple cider vinegar every day, we've discovered that it brings a healthy, rosy glow to one's complexion! This is great news if you suffer from a pale countenance.

What to Expect from this Book

Over the years we have come to love and cherish our online community. It has made us part of a group that has brought so much health and real happiness to people all over the world, as well as freedom from pain and relief from the anxiety about health when health is lacking. That's exactly as much as we could ask from life. We are very proud of EarthClinic.com, but the internet can't be with us everywhere, not on Grandma's farm when Johnny's allergies start up or out at camp when Rebekkah feels sick to her stomach from eating too many roasted marshmallows. We'd also like to welcome all the folks into our community who wouldn't know an internet if it zapped them in the USB port!

This book has been woven together with those ideas in mind, for those people who want to keep the secrets of ACV close at home even if a computer is far away, the loyal community members who want to share our secrets with friends and family, and for the people who would never meet up with these ideas unless they were to be found on a book rack or a coffee table.

If you have visited our website, much of this will be familiar to you. We have distilled the best and most informative feedback about ACV from that invaluable resource, but there is much you will find that is new as well. Earth Clinic trusts in the voice of personal experience and has let that voice do most of the talking on the website, but now we want to support all of those personal reports (yes, you'll find the best of them in here) with a bit of history and the reassuring certainty that scientific study can offer.

Chapter 2

APPLE CIDER VINEGAR: A CLASSIC REMEDY

Apple cider vinegar is quite unlike this continuing parade of miracle cures we've seen and read so much about of late. It isn't one of those cure-alls that strut briefly to their spot in front of the global grandstand, soon to depart after a moment of fame. ACV has been a cure for what ails you for as long as there has been any sort of medicine at all. The use of vinegar in general is as old as human history; wherever there have been alcoholic beverages, some form of vinegar was sure to follow, and at least the most obvious virtues and exotic allure of vinegar would have been recognized right away.

Of course, that begs the question as to why a book such as this need even exist. If vinegar has been around for that long, shouldn't the world have come to appreciate it by now? By and large, the answer is yes, and the reason there is a need for this book is simply that we have forgotten all of its virtues and erased the once worthy role of vinegars from our life. Certainly, we still have vinegar here and there in the course of our diets, such as they are, but modern grocery stores and the international food trade offer us so many choices that foundational parts of our historical diets, such as vinegar once was, have been pushed aside for mere variety (or, more regrettably, for the easy pleasure of fast food and junk foods).

Clearly something isn't right. This should be the age of medical miracles, but our health complaints seem to be at an all time high. There you have the other reason why this book has a necessary place in the world. Take for instance acid reflux and similar digestive disorders, which seem to affect everyone these days. Few people would think to add an acid like ACV to their diet to bring relief from an acid condition, yet our readers are astounded by their success in using ACV to permanently settle their acid reflux and heartburn. The half dozen producers of expensive commercial medicines targeting acid reflux would hardly be pleased to have us consider a natural, inexpensive alternative. But it works!

HIPPOCRATES

Despite the many years that have passed between then and now, today's health care and medical fields perhaps have never so much resembled any other period in history as the era when medicine was first truly born—with Hippocrates in ancient Greece. At Earth Clinic, we try to reconcile the wisdom of folk medicine with the wonders of modern science. Similarly, Hippocrates created Western medicine in his efforts to bring a scientific method to practical ideas about food and the body that were prevalent in his time.

Hippocrates lived between 460 and 370 BC, in the wondrous Age of Pericles. It is after him that the Hippocratic Oath was named, the promise modern doctors still make to "first, do no harm" when entering into their medical careers.

Ironically, much that is said to be true about Hippocrates is likely myth or the work of other hands. Even the Hippocratic Oath was most likely written by another author. The irony is that Hippocrates was truly the first practitioner of clinical medicine, looking at the signs and symptoms that appeared in the patient's body and behavior to diagnose the underlying problems that ailed that patient. Physicians from the Hippocratic School took case histories and respected the importance of cleanliness in how and where they treated patients, just as our doctors do today. Hippocrates and his students drew the world away from the common belief that illnesses were judgments from the gods. Instead, he looked as we do for specific changes in the body and in our environments that could lead to illness, and in finding them he would then apply remedies that would counteract those influences and re-balance the body.

Among his most common prescriptions was for the use of oxymel, a combination of vinegar and honey that he thought would balance the four humours (black and yellow bile, blood, and phlegm) in a patient's body. Today we know those humours don't function in the body as Hippocrates thought, yet we still enjoy the benefits of apple cider vinegar and honey in knowing that their enzymes, vitamins, and minerals will help restore that same systemic balance that Hippocrates was seeking when he prescribed it 2400 years ago.

The success of modern science has been so remarkable — a fact we admit and enjoy ourselves — that we have entirely given up the gems of knowledge our ancestors dug up through centuries of trial and error. The wonders of modern medical science still leave us with massive gaps in our knowledge of human health and wellness, and many of those holes can be filled with old folk wisdom.

We need a renaissance in health that restores our ability to value and use our inherited medical knowledge, creating a realm of modern folk medicine. As for Earth Clinic, we want to be a part of that, and we're going to start with apple cider vinegar.

History of the Apple

Starting with apple cider vinegar actually requires us to take a few steps further back to where vinegar comes from. Unlike your simple apple or beefsteak, vinegar is a third generation food in that it takes two precursor steps to reach the ACV endpoint — acetification that forms the vinegar itself, and before that the fermentation of apple cider to create the alcohol molecules that will be converted into acetic acid. So before we ever get to talk about the production and use of apple cider vinegar, we need to talk a bit about the history and virtues of alcoholic or hard apple cider and of course about apples themselves.

As ubiquitous and widespread as the apple is in countries throughout the world, the trees that produce eating apples would be quite an isolated species of plant were it not for the eager work of human hands. Our US readers who consider apples and apple pie as near to the core of American identity as Mom and the Bill of Rights might be surprised to learn that 'eating apples' and 'cider apples' are not native to any part of the country, although the fruit tree appeared on the continent nearly as early as the first European settlers.

The only apple tree native to North America is the crabapple, a separate species in the same genus. Nevertheless, it can cross-fertilize with cider and sweet apple trees just as well.

As a tree belonging to the rose or *Rosaceae* family, the apple tree genus has a single commercial species *Malus domestica*, but an ever-increasing number of cultivars (cultivated varieties) that already number over 7500. Those cultivars were carefully transplanted, cross-pollinated, and grafted ever further from their origins in the mountains of eastern Kazakhstan through ten thousand years of human cultivation. Persia and then Iran became tremendous producers and partakers in apples, and the fruit took tremendous hold in China as well, where much of the country is particularly well suited to the apple tree. In the West, Persians passed along apple nursery practices to European traders. Those practices were taken up by the Romans who carried apple trees with them throughout Europe and into England, which in many ways has become the international heart of apple cultivation.

> *The apple tree originated in an area of Central Asia between the Black Sea and the Caspian. It was one of the first trees to come under human cultivation and has since been carried all across the world.*

This profusion of apple culture, together with and resulting from the apple's plentiful gifts in flavor and nutrition, make it no wonder that apples have become synonymous with virtue and beauty — as well as with great temptation — in cultures throughout the world. From the Garden of Eden to the virtuous gentlemen William Tell and Johnny Appleseed and through Snow White's wicked queen the apple has spread throughout religious stories and social mythology. Even in scientific mythology, with the fall of Newton's apple and the discovery of gravity, there has been an abundance of attention directed toward the apple orchard, with justifiable reason.

From England this love of the apple was broadcast to the Americas. The history of apple cider vinegar in the United States begins with the introduction of apples to the colonies by English colonists — the very Pilgrims themselves. While crab apples were indigenous to the area, they seem to have been little used, but once eating and cider apples were introduced to the Massachusetts Bay Colony, first brought over on later voyages of the Mayflower, they soon spread throughout the continent. In particular, the legendary Johnny Appleseed spread apple trees and apple culture westward, but he was hardly alone.

Apples were justly prized as both a pleasure and as an essential, with winter apples carrying a family through the hard winter. Without fresh food available in the months following the last harvest, settlers had to count on apples. Apples kept well for later eating, produced cider and hard cider for refreshment, and provided apple cider vinegar to help pickle and preserve the autumn harvest for later consumption.

JOHNNY APPLESEED

The legendary Johnny Appleseed was born as John Chapman in 1774, a perfectly ordinary young man who grew up the son of a poor farmer in Leominster, Massachusetts. His father had him apprenticed as a nurseryman in a neighbor's apple orchard, and from that training and a firm belief in the practical and symbolic virtues of the apple, Johnny Appleseed was figuratively born.

Even while he was alive, Chapman was growing into the legend he would eventually become, largely thanks to his genial good nature and pleasant oddities—the image of him traveling with only a sack of seeds and seedlings, wearing a coffee sack as a shirt and a stove pot as a hat, while not literally true, is probably not so far from the truth. Chapman set out westward from Massachusetts when he was 18, continuing on intermittently and making summertime circuits in all directions, eventually planting apple trees throughout Ohio, Illinois, and Indiana.

While a particularly Christian man and a missionary for the Swedenborgian Church of the New Jerusalem, Chapman was also a more talented businessman than he is typically given credit for. Granted, he was a businessman inclined to forget and to forgive debts that were owed him. Part of his legendary image comes from the fact that he would accept used clothing as payment and would wear the worst of the clothing in his possession at all times until it became useless.

Chapman ran what we would call a franchise business, setting up apple tree nurseries just ahead of the waves of westward American expansion. All along the paths of his travels, he would share the profits from the sale of his nursery stock with the local farmer who tended those trees.

To our particular delight and pleasure, most of Chapman's apple trees were of the cider variety.

Chapman passed away in 1845 in his adopted home of Fort Wayne, Indiana where he had hundreds of acres of farmland dedicated to apple growing and apple seedling cultivation for sale to other farmers throughout the country. Yet his success in business was quickly forgotten, paling in comparison to his success in bringing laughter with him in all his travels, and in being at peace within every settler's cabin, in forest or field, and between the villages of Native Americans and European settlers alike.

Apples into Cider: Sweet and Hard

The many uses of apples were hardly first discovered in the American colonies. In fact it seems that Aryan tribes of the Near East first developed a version of hard cider as a popular drink around 2500 BC, a drink the Phoenicians later called "shekar" and passed along to later cultures such as the Greeks. The Romans under Julius Caesar found alcoholic cider to be a popular drink among the Celts they were attempting to conquer in England, showing how widely apples and apple juices had traveled by the time of Christ. Thus while Charlemagne was conquering Europe in the name of the Christian God, he was also finding it important to create laws regulating and taxing the cider industry of the time.

For many centuries in Europe, apple cider in both sweet and hard varieties was among the most common of drinks, even to the point where it was often used as currency to pay taxes and debts. Cider was for centuries much more popular than either wine or beer, and often safer than simple water. In pre-modern cities the drinking water was often contaminated and dangerous to one's health — threats that were minimized by fruit juices and eliminated by the alcohol in fermented beverages.

Thus was much effort put into apple cider production, where again we begin with the apples themselves. As there are apples best for fresh eating and for baking, there are cider apples that produce better cider than would be made from dessert apples. Cider apples are more tart, generally too tart for eating, but that sharp flavor mellows out in the fermentation and aging processes to give apple cider its broad flavor. However, those cider apples are often mixed with sweet apples for a sugary appeal.

Nearly forty apples go into each gallon of apple cider.

Beyond selecting the proper blend of apples, a balance that cider makers take as seriously as others do in evaluating wine grapes, the process of making apple cider is a more or less straightforward process of squishing and filtering. Nevertheless, there are degrees, variations, and distinctions beginning with the difference between apple juice and apple cider. Apple juicing methods are approximately the same for both drinks, but apple cider is less thoroughly processed and filtered, leaving behind more of the nutrients and biotic materials that we value nutritionally. You should be able to see some of those unfiltered solids as a cloudy suspension that gives apple cider its characteristically dark color. Ideally, apple cider is also unpasteurized, though it is difficult to find unpasteurized apple cider these days unless directly from local orchards.

Typically, apple cider is produced on site at an apple orchard, whereas apple juice is liable to be more of a factory operation, with apples often shipped a great distance to a facility that industrially processes the apples of a number of orchards for the broader consumer market. Conversely, your apple cider may have been squeezed out by more or less the same apple cider press that has been in use on a family farm for several generations. Modern machinery is more efficient and thorough, but typically it takes 10-15 pounds of apples to make one gallon of cider, regardless of the mechanism.

The process of making apple cider is not entirely simple, but the basic steps include collection of a large number of apples, sometimes including 'drops', which are the healthy apples that have dropped off their trees at the peak of ripeness. Those apples are then cleaned and cut or macerated into what is more or less uncooked applesauce, except that the sauce contains every bit of the apple, from skin to seeds. While you may not be a fan of apple skins, and very few of us eat the seeds, you may well be familiar with the fact that fruit skins are often the best sources of nutrients and fiber out of the entire fruit, and seeds of all sorts are always of necessity packed full of energy and nutrition. They have to give birth to entire trees, after all.

That complete apple mash is then wrapped in cheesecloth or another porous filter and then with a cider press is thoroughly squeezed of all its apple juices. If the term 'cider mill' rings a bell, this is a machine that in one mechanism combines the pressing process with the chopping and grinding first step.

Stringent filtering and thorough pasteurization of the resulting apple cider significantly extends the shelf life of what consequently becomes apple juice. That shelf life has helped it to become a favorite of parents and children everywhere. However, the processing also kills off the yeasts that would naturally begin to transform apple cider into hard apple cider given time. Otherwise, pure sweet cider will naturally turn into hard cider, whether intentionally or when you have left the cider too long in the back of your refrigerator.

While Canada and the United States make a distinction between hard cider and sweet or soft cider, in much of the world the term 'cider' refers only to that fermented version of apple drinks created by time and those naturally occurring yeasts. Just as in the process of leavening, where yeast (a microscopic fungus that can be found anywhere you choose to look for it) converts sugars into the carbon dioxide that causes bread to rise, yeast will also create alcohol as a byproduct of digesting sugars. The sweet delights of cider offer sugars aplenty for naturally occurring yeasts to act on, adding bubbly carbon dioxide and alcohol molecules to create hard or alcoholic cider with or without the help of apple cider makers. And there ends the first part of our cider vinegar making tale.

Too often, illnesses and imbalances in our bodies are the fault of parasitic viruses, germs, and bacteria entering our systems. Ironically, the blessings of apple cider vinegar are the product of two families of fungus and bacteria that go to work on apple cider to create ACV's regenerative properties. Yeast of the genus Saccharomyces catalyze the first fermentation of cider into hard cider, while bacteria in the acetobacter family transition the alcohol produced in the first fermentation process into acetic acid, the basis of vinegar, while also producing other nutritious compounds.

The Life and Times of Vinegar

Vinegar was presumably never so much discovered as it came to be appreciated as something of value. Humanity didn't have to invent vinegar, it comes along on its own through the natural acetification of all sorts of fruit juices and other sugary liquids that are left out long enough — to first become alcoholic and then become converted into vinegar. Both of these are natural and more or less inevitable processes that would have occurred on their own over and over again before anyone learned to enjoy them. Though to be sure, our ancestors no doubt grew to appreciate the conversion of sugars into alcohol more or less immediately, no matter how little they understood the process at the outset.

Alcohol, when it formed naturally and more or less accidentally, would have done then as it does now, seduce us quite readily and pleasurably. Thereafter, any of those alcoholic drinks that were left exposed to air for a bit longer would have made the transition to vinegar. At first people were liable to think of that transformation as a loss, ruining the wine or grain alcohol they had labored to produce. Only slowly, you would imagine, would people have come to appreciate vinegar's preservative usefulness and then the delectable virtues of vinegar's challenging, even dangerous-seeming flavor.

Babylonian accounts in 5000 BC are the first known written record of any form of vinegar, that particular vinegar having been made from the juice of the date palm. Yet by 400 BC, Hippocrates, the father of medicine, was prescribing it for everything from rheumatism to congestion. Hippocrates was particularly fond of a combination of vinegar and honey, which was called oxymel.

He was far from alone in savoring its virtues. Throughout the world cultures have transformed the handiest available sugar sources into vinegars of all strengths and flavors, including rice vinegar; vinegars from any numbers of fruits including raspberries and coconuts; sugar vinegars derived from honey, molasses, and maple syrup; and vegetable vinegars like you can get from the juice of beets. Among common alcoholic drinks, it is not only rice and grape wines that join hard cider as vinegar sources, but beer vinegar is also available (malt vinegar more or less deriving from beer as well) and in Mexico you can find tequila vinegar.

From all this diversity, we can conclude that vinegar production developed separately many times throughout the world, and its healthy properties were likewise no doubt repeatedly uncovered by intellectuals and concerned mothers alike. Vinegar was used as a tonic for strength by Japanese samurai, sailors throughout the world and history combated scurvy with apple cider vinegar, soldiers in the Civil War and the First World War used it to clean wounds, while English and American farmers brought vinegar beverages out into the fields to help them carry on beneath the hot midday sun. Readers of the Bible may have thought that it was a further insult when soldiers offered Christ a sponge full of vinegar and water while on the cross, but in fact Roman soldiers often used diluted vinegar as a fortifying drink for themselves on long marches.

The potency of vinegar is highlighted by two famous stories that practically mythologize vinegar's virtues. In the first, Cleopatra was said to have dissolved a string of pearls in a glass of vinegar (a feat that has been tested and found to be true) which she then drank to win a bet she had made with Marc Antony that she could eat a meal of astronomical cost at a single seating. The second tale concerns the great general Hannibal, who was said to have used fire and vinegar alone to crack and dissolve massive boulders that stood in the mountain paths of his army and its elephants on their way into Italy against the Romans.

It was through the Romans that apple cider and then apple cider vinegar first came into the historical record, when Julius Caesar's Roman Legions began to conquer the Gallic tribes of England, where hard apple cider was very popular. Thereafter, apple cider and vinegar both spread across Europe and throughout history. As it spread in Europe, vinegar eventually earned its modern name from the Old French term *vin aigre*, which meant "sour wine", a very literal description of wine turned sour by acetic acid.

Acetic Acid is a weak acid, formally known as ethanoic acid, formed by acetobacter bacteria. It gives every type of vinegar its sour flavor and typical odor. In the body, acetic acid plays an important role in metabolizing both fats and carbohydrates.

Alongside the expansion of vinegar as a food ingredient and preservative, as well as in preserving health, vinegar also enjoyed a continual evolution in the way it was produced. Nature laid the path for producing basic vinegars of all sorts, but as is often the case with the works of Nature, people have done their best to improve on natural vinegar. In part, this was simply the continued effort to experiment with different raw materials for vinegars. Beyond ingredients, however, there was also the process used for creating vinegar that could be tinkered with, and several processes developed, each with their own virtues.

In terms of quality, the best way to produce any sort of vinegar is to do it slowly. Modern methods, on the other hand, accelerate the process as much as possible through the use of aeration tanks. Far preferable to that system of mass production is the Orleans Process, which has been used to produce vinegar since its formulation in Orleans, France in 1394, during the Middle Ages. Created by a group of French winemakers eager to turn the misfortune of soured wine into the bounty of a market for culinary vinegar, the Orleans Process sought to bring the same richness and depth of flavor to vinegar as French vintners had created in their wines.

The process uses the same sorts of wooden casks as are used to age fine wines. The cask is turned on its side and has holes drilled into both ends of the barrel about three-quarters of the way to the top. Hard cider (or another vinegar-making alcoholic liquid) is poured into the cask up to that line, and cheesecloth or another mesh is placed over the holes to keep insects and dust out of the maturing vinegar. In this way, the hard apple cider is exposed to the air over the largest possible surface area; this is important since the acid forming acetobacter bacteria need oxygen to transform the alcohol molecules.

Acetobacter is the genus of bacteria responsible for the transformation of the alcohol in fermented apple cider into the acetic acid of apple cider vinegar. Acetobacter bacteria are present in the air and naturally find their way to any alcohol compounds, but they can also be introduced in the process of creating ACV.

Modern vinegar-making methods simply produce acetic acid. However, the Orleans Process extends the work of the vinegar-making bacteria over several weeks, allowing the vinegar and its components to fully mature. Then the developed vinegar is allowed to sit for another year or more and age just as a wine would. This allows the vinegar to develop more complicated flavors and reduces its acidic bite. It also provides time enough for the basic constituents of the vinegar to further develop into all the beneficial enzymes and nutraceuticals that make apple cider vinegar as potent a health agent as it can be.

Complex foods are generally more flavorful and enjoyable, but more importantly they tend to be more full of healthy components. When we cook a meal or otherwise produce some sort of food, its complexity comes from using the best raw materials and the most patient techniques. This is as true for creating wine or vinegar as it is for making the perfect soufflé. In the case of apple cider vinegar in particular, the ideal process begins with cider made from whole apples mashed into a pulp and cold-pressed. That cider should then be stored and fermented in wood barrels to draw out vinegar of the best quality. In that way, you get apple cider vinegar with all the same nutrients you look for when you bite into an apple. In particular, you have potassium, but you also have flavonoids, and beta-carotene (Vitamin A), which are powerful antioxidants, sweeping up the dangerous free radicals in our bodies and thereby preventing cancer. Apples also offer pectin, the soluble fiber that figures in jams and jellies. Add to all of that the work of the fermentation process, which produces many additional enzymes and amino acids not present in the apple itself.

There are of course many other techniques for creating vinegar, including methods that are simple enough for the kitchen counter. Modern vinegar factories use aeration in vast tanks of apple cider or another raw material, turning the liquid over repeatedly and adding needed oxygen to speed up the work of the acetobacter strains in creating acetic acid. Yet you can make your own ACV in a crockpot.

Back at the other end of the scale, the Solera Method is the slowest way to produce vinegar, and some will say that it produces the most delightful, complicated, and health-promoting vinegars. The finest vintages of wine are in fact reserved for the Solera Method, creating wine vinegars priced as expensively as fine wines would be, and the method can be used on apple cider as well.

It's sort of remarkable how complicated we can make the process of creating vinegar, when it is a transformation that would naturally happen on its own. It's also sort of amusing that as it is an apple's sugars that are converted into alcohol and then into acetic acid, sweeter apples will produce more acidic vinegar. There are many such interesting ironies to apple cider vinegar — the antibacterial cleanser produced by bacteria, the acid that can remedy acid-reflux, and ACV the acid that can produce an alkaline reaction in the body.

And all of that is not to mention the fact that we're cheering the health benefits of a "wonder drug" that you can find in the grocery store stocked between the ketchup and the mayonnaise! Why should we invest such effort in something so ordinary, and how in the world is it liable to do us all that much good? There are two categories of answer to that question: the complicated but more or less straightforward answer, and the nitty-gritty science of apple cider vinegar. We will try to offer you both, beginning with everyday facts you need.

The problem with aphorisms like "An apple a day keeps the doctor away" is that repetition makes the truth seem stale and of doubtful value. How about this for a fresh, modern rendition of the old wisdom: "An apple full of boron and minerals for bones, polyphenols and flavonoids to fight free radicals, enzymes and soluble fiber to help the digestive system, acid to fight infections, and a host of vitamins a day keeps the doctor away." Not quite as bite-sized, but just as true!

Why It's the Good Stuff

Modern medicine is constantly in search of the single answer to all of our medical problems. After all, scientists have delivered us remarkable blessings, and that great history of success and promise has us ever hoping for the silver bullet that will kill cancer, the silver bullet to defeat HIV/AIDS, the silver bullet against the wide complex of syndromes that constitute heart disease. Unfortunately, just as with the true horrors that inspire simple fables like the werewolf, the human body is much more complicated. Silver bullets kill mythical beasts in stories, but in real life we need to address the complexity of reality with our own complex answers to life's problems — including issues with our health.

Apple cider vinegar is not a silver bullet, a panacea, or cure-all. Nevertheless, it has great virtue, and that value lies in its complexity. ACV contributes to all the major activities of the body: digestion, circulation, activity, maintenance, and construction. Carbohydrates and enzymes in ACV support the body's energy-making systems. Potassium and acids smooth the flow of blood through the veins and of water and nutrients between those veins and the body's cells. ACV's acids help in digestion, as do certain of its enzymes. Its proteins go to building new cells and both its acidic and alkalizing properties help to maintain the body's homeostasis.

The components of unfiltered apple cider vinegar are principally water and leftover solids that get through the minimal filtration process from the cider press. However, it is the array of minerals, enzymes, and acids in apple cider vinegar that are of most interest to us. Acetic acid (the vinegar acid) is the most plentiful of these components. After that, we find various forms of sugar, mineral ash, tannins, protein (mostly valuable enzymes), calcium phosphate, potassium, sodium, iron, zinc, riboflavin, and traces of other elements. Apple cider vinegar is very much like the multivitamins sold to us by the storefull, but in a form that the body recognizes and can immediately absorb.

As to ACV's vinegar components, they shouldn't be dismissed as merely an interesting flavor. While it's little talked about, our bodies seem to crave vinegar because the body knows what it needs (in the way that pregnant women crave pickles, and not so much in the way that we crave rocky road ice cream at midnight). In addition to acetic acid, ACV also typically contains malic acid, ascorbic acid, and lactic acid.

Medical research has confirmed what people have known for centuries, that thanks to these acid components, ACV kills bacteria (including gram-negative bacteria) and other microorganisms. However, scientific studies also offer confirmation that ACV kills bacteria inside of our bodies even once we have consumed apple cider vinegar, which is a benefit not as easily proven outside of the lab.

Furthermore, studies have proven that apple cider vinegar can help in breaking down drugs in the body, detoxifying our systems by making it easy for us to excrete those drugs and chemicals. Acids, by their very nature, are bactericidal and germicidal. Most living things simply do not endure an acidic environment very easily. Large organisms like ourselves can handle and even make use of a bit of acid, but single-celled pathogens are quickly dissolved or denatured in the presence of a solvent like the acetic acid in vinegar.

Bacteria are simply another form of life, akin to the broad categories of plants and animals. They are absolutely everywhere, are single-celled and therefore microscopically small, and as with the rest of life on earth, some of them are good for us, some bad, and most have nothing to do with human life whatsoever. For each Mycobacterium tuberculosis that causes tuberculosis, there is an acetic acid bacterium to add flavor and nutrition to our lives.

Brands of ACV

Forgive us if we put the apple cart before the horse here, but this would be a good moment to talk about the differences between brands and kinds of ACV. As far as brands go, well that'll be quick. Earth Clinic tries to stay as impartial as we can be, and for certain we never accept payments or considerations from any companies in order to support their products. The most we'll say about ACV brands then is that the more famous the name on the bottle, the more likely you are to be disappointed. Major brands tend to use simple white vinegar with apple flavoring. It's cheaper for them, but it isn't the real stuff with all the benefits we have found in honest to goodness ACV.

There are, in fact, fairly few respectable options out there for genuine apple cider vinegar. You may have to travel around a bit before you find the grocery, country, or health food store that offers the good stuff. Of course, the internet does offer several options where you can place an order and have it delivered to your home. When you do go out in search of a good bottle of ACV, keep your eyes open for hints on the label and the ingredients list. There should be only the one ingredient.

In particular, you might find a label on a bottle of ACV that says something about "the Mother", which sounds a bit odd. What that label is talking about though is something we rather like, grainy remains you'll find settled to the bottom of the bottle, remnants of the raw materials from which the ACV was originally brewed. "The Mother" is proof positive that what you have in your hands is the genuine article and probably the bottle you want to go home with.

Mother of Vinegar, or "the Mother", is the floating mass of acetobacter xylinum found at the top of an active batch of apple cider vinegar. This island of bacteria creates your acetic acid. The Mother can be transferred to new batches of hard apple cider to start the vinegar-making process. It produces strands of cellulose that you can see dropping down from the floating island of the Mother.

Types of Vinegar

Clearly, apple cider vinegar is not the only sort of vinegar available. Vinegar, in fact, varies remarkably and can be found with regional variations throughout the world. Even when distilled from the same basic components, like grapes and rice, vinegar is often infused with herbs and flavorful ingredients like peppers and garlic, expanding the diversity of vinegar options even more.

It is primarily a vinegar's principle ingredient that determines its quality and characteristics, whether that be apples, rice, grapes, or what have you. The basic production of vinegar does not vary significantly. In every case, some base ingredient is processed into a liquid form, fermented, and then allowed to transform into vinegar. Any one of these vinegars could then be heated and condensed to produce distilled vinegar — a nearly pure combination of water and acetic acid (5-8% concentration) that you commonly find in the grocery store. Distilled vinegar is great for cleaning and the like, but nearly useless for our health, since the process of distillation eliminates all the vitamins, minerals, and enzymes from the mix.

There are also synthetic vinegars, actually produced from petroleum derivatives or coal tar, which produces vinegar as little good for your health as it is pleasant to think about. The thought of vinegar from a barrel of petroleum or a lump of coal is a bit disgusting, and hardly likely to instill much confidence as a source of health.

Imitation vinegar can mimic apple cider vinegar and other flavorful vinegars by taking basic distilled vinegar and adding flavorings to match the intended product. While that can be perfectly suitable for adding (artificial) flavors to cooking, it doesn't offer nearly the health benefits of the original. You will want to pay attention to this point, as many of the widely available commercial apple cider vinegars are exactly this sort of imitation vinegar, rather than the good stuff, the stuff we in the Earth Clinic community look for ourselves.

Still, all of these vinegars, the better and the worse, add flavor to food, can kill germs and bacteria, and may have some positive health benefits when it comes to cancers, obesity, cholesterol levels, and perhaps other areas of health and beauty. Then why is it that we prefer apple cider vinegar to other vinegar candidates? Well, we certainly wouldn't want to dismiss the virtues of other vinegars. Red wine vinegar in particular has deserved much recent notice as a cancer fighter and general health tonic.

Still, we prefer ACV to the others for a number of reasons, starting with the greater nutritive value of apples themselves. The apple is the source of all the complexity ACV offers, a whole array of vitamins, minerals, and enzymes. Likewise, ACV is more versatile in the kitchen than other vinegars.

Apples are free of sodium, fat, and cholesterol.

Yet when it comes down to specifics, ACV is the vinegar of choice because of two definite characteristics: its high levels of potassium and its ability to restore the body's pH balance to a more alkaline level.

Let's deal with the second and more complicated topic first. We all vaguely recall the concepts of acids and bases/alkalis from high school science classes, and you may also remember that few creatures like very acidic or very alkaline environments. Our own bodies prefer just the same, a life neither too acidic nor too basic. However, different parts of our bodies — the skin, our blood, the internal organs, the insides of our digestive systems, and our cells themselves — each prefer different environments, some slightly or even significantly acidic (the inside of the stomach, where digestion occurs) and other organs prefer a more alkaline or basic environment. Maintaining that balance within one body requires a number of biological mechanisms to help keep the body functioning well and happily.

Taken as a complete food, ACV is an acid that nevertheless alkalizes (makes more basic) the bloodstream and through it the body as a whole. This may quite understandably be confusing at first. In fact, it is an area that welcomes plenty of argument and confusion even within the apple cider vinegar community. Yet it is just as obvious that no food goes straight into our bodies and through the stomach to the bloodstream without alteration.

Foods are processed in the stomach and intestines, so that it isn't acetic acid that necessarily reaches our blood but all the metabolized parts of ACV, as with all our foods. In the case of apple cider vinegar, the most important component reaching our bloodstream is potassium. ACV is full of it, offering 240 milligrams of potassium per cup, and the mineral turns out to be an important alkalizing mineral, one that we are often deficient in through the course of our normal diets.

And so it turns out that the two most important characteristics of ACV come down more or less to one and the same thing. Potassium, however, plays more than just an alkalizing role in maintaining our health. Potassium's role in our bodies is all about movement and balance, which are each as essential to our cells and organs as to our daily lives as a complete organism. The potassium in our bodies is found almost entirely within our cells, just as almost all of the body's salt is to be found in the bloodstream, and the dance between those two positively charged mineral ions is what keeps just enough fluid inside of our cells, while needed nutrients flow into those cells and wastes flow out. Salt and potassium also play a key role in nerve function, creating the electrical potential energy needed to send signals across our nerve endings. Perhaps most important of all, those two minerals together are essential to proper muscle functioning, including the muscles of the heart.

> *Potassium is a relatively common element and alkali metal found in the form of ionic salts in nature and as an essential mineral ion in all plants and animals. As the other half of the sodium-potassium pump that regulates water retention and flow between and within the cells of the body, potassium helps to regulate the flow of nutrients, wastes, and electrical signals throughout the body.*

Our health can't be simplified down to only these two mineral components, but our modern diets have undergone such a radical change from what our chemical systems were built to accommodate that it has begun to cause dramatic symptoms of general ill health. Ideally, the ratio of potassium to sodium in our diets would be 5:1. That is in line with the relative unavailability of sodium and the plenitude of potassium in normal plant-based diets, the sort of meals our bodies over millennia were built to enjoy. Yet these days, sodium typically enters our diets at levels twice that of potassium.

Too much salt in our diet. We've all heard the refrain before, but that imbalance leads to shortages of what the body needs, and it requires that we exert extra effort in order to force our systems into a relative balance, a balance that should come more naturally. The potassium in ACV helps to level out our intense consumption of salt in modern diets. Thanks to an absence of sodium and its generous share of potassium, ACV can do much to restore the proper ratio and bring balance to cardiac functioning and all the potassium-sodium mechanisms operating in the body.

That imbalance between the potassium our bodies need and the sodium it is being overwhelmed by goes a long way to explain the epidemic of fatigue, muscle weakness, headaches, muscle aches, irritability, skin conditions and mental fuzziness that many of us suffer from. ACV can play a pivotal role in bringing that imbalance back to normal and restore us to healthier lives.

Yet in perfect truth, the amount of potassium in apple cider vinegar cannot make up for the total shortage of potassium we find in our typical diets. It is an excellent supplement, but without other changes in your eating habits, particularly to include more fruit and vegetable servings, your potassium deficit can't be made up. Thus it stands to reason that the genuine benefits so many people have found in apple cider vinegar cannot be attributed to potassium alone, although many have tried. Potassium was the key interest of Dr. Jarvis in his study of apple cider vinegar, so the appreciation for this micronutrient is well placed, but it cannot explain the value of ACV all on its own. Which is why we again return to the natural complexity of all those components we are offered in ACV, and in particular to the complex phytochemicals created in the vinegar-making process. Most of these plant chemicals have gone almost completely unstudied, but new revelations about the benefits our bodies derive from those still mysterious products of fruits and vegetables are uncovered all the time.

All of this merely serves as an introduction to the medical benefits offered by ACV. The next chapter goes into more detail on how ACV fills holes in our diet and offers information from the most recent scientific investigations into ACV as a health supplement. However, we stand by the belief that it is the direct feedback on ACV cures that we have gotten from our readers that best argues for its effectiveness. Therefore, if you are already convinced that apple cider vinegar is something worth checking out, or if you simply want to leap into the heart of the matter, feel free to skip ahead to Chapter Four and our explanations of which conditions can be addressed through the multiple uses of apple cider vinegar, together with first person accounts of how those remedies have worked for people around the world. Otherwise, the bell is about to ring for science class.

D.C. JARVIS, M.D.

D.C. Jarvis, M.D. is in many ways the forefather of what we would call modern folk medicine. His book, Folk Medicine: A Vermont Country Doctor's Guide to Good Health, was intended only as a collection of Doctor Jarvis' findings, to be passed down to his daughter and their descendants. Yet it found its way into a publisher's hands and has since become a classic of medical literature and in particular a cornerstone of folk medicine.

Through the book and his research, Dr. Jarvis brought ancient wisdom into a modern context. As a Vermonter, a man of the countryside, and as a rural doctor he brought modern medical rigor and the scientific process to bear on ages of earned folk wisdom.

Born in Plattsburg, NY on March 15, 1881, DeForest Clinton Jarvis grew up in Burlington, Vermont and studied medicine at the University of Vermont Medical College on his way to a career as an otolaryngologist and ophthalmologist with a practice in Barre, Vermont. His curiosity, studies, and his deep and friendly concern for his patients were the key ingredients that opened up the world of folk medicine to a wider audience. His scientific examination of those traditional treatments he learned from his patients was expanded by his habit of looking to the animal world to find what all life held in common, in particular examining dairy herds with an eye towards the health concerns involved in safe and optimal milk production.

Folk Medicine has sold over a million copies and has been in print since its publication in 1958. Dr. Jarvis passed away in 1966 at the age of 85.

Dr. Jarvis would have been the last man to deny the wonders of modern medicine and science in general. However, he found it just as foolish to entirely abandon the medical wisdom of the hard-fought past, not while modern medical treatments are still puzzling out the complexity of human life. While modern science produces miracles that lengthen and improve our lives, it is still a young discipline given to the egotistical blunders of youth. Doctor Jarvis was eager for modern cures, but he relied on traditional medicines like kelp, honey, seafood, and apple cider vinegar to maintain our daily health in the meantime.

Chapter 3

THE SCIENCE OF APPLE CIDER VINEGAR

Much of the science in the previous chapter should have been a bit familiar, sticking to the same nutritional information we hear everyday. Newspapers and nutritionists drill these same concepts about fiber, nutrients, and all the rest into our heads, trying to help us in choosing the best foods for our long-term health. Some of it we hear and remember, some of it goes over our heads, and sometimes the experts change their minds so many times that we just don't pay attention. Vinegar in general and apple cider vinegar specifically, on the other hand, are here to stay and have been in use for centuries. So if you would like a more complete explanation of the science behind apple cider vinegar and its benefits, we will take a look at why it works and what ACV can offer. And we'll make it as little like Mrs. Grozner's sophomore biology class as possible, promise!

Unfortunately, we have to begin with the caveat that, in fact, there are many questions about the virtues of ACV that we cannot answer. Science has largely given up on studying topics as common and inexpensive as vinegar. Scientific and medical research is big business, and as that research is often expensive, researchers direct almost all of their studies to medicines that can be sold for billions rather than everyday home remedies that can be sold at the grocery store.

Fortunately, we don't have to know how it works to know that it works. As an illustration of that fact, we can look back at one of the more famous anecdotes about the life preserving properties of vinegar, a story that dates back to the Black Plague, in an equally black tale. It seems a group of thieves was having remarkable luck in both loot and survival through a series of thefts against houses that were sick with the plague — houses that no one else dared enter, not even caregivers. When they were at last caught, the thieves ascribed their success and survival to apple cider vinegar. In the interest of public safety, the thieves were allowed to escape the gallows by offering up their antibiotic formulation, which they would repeatedly wash their bodies with, and which became known as the Four Thieves Vinegar Formula.

Four Thieves Vinegar

- *3 Quarts ACV*
- *3 Tablespoons each rosemary, lavender, sage, mint, rue, and plantain*
- *6 cloves garlic*
- *Combine and allow to sit uncovered for 24 hours before use*

The Four Thieves Vinegar recipe can be used as a cleansing and disinfecting agent for hard surfaces, and with care it can even be ingested a teaspoon at a time to fight viruses.

Of course, this was in an age long before the understanding offered by modern medicine, much less any knowledge of viruses or just what it was that the Four Thieves Vinegar recipe was protecting anyone against. Nevertheless, the thieves survived because whatever science was behind the ACV, it did its job whether or not they understood the source of their luck.

Still, now that a better understanding is available we should make an effort to get a grasp on the science. To start off, let's look into the concept of acidity.

The Acid/Alkaline Balance

Our bodies are always looking to maintain homeostasis — the condition of balance throughout all the body's mechanisms and constituent parts. In that way, our physical bodies are much like our psychological and social selves, we want most of the things around us to be dependable and constant. A little bit of variation or thrill is probably just as welcome to our bodies as it is in our lives, but altogether we want life to be predictable. While every now and again it's good for us to do something daring, we want to have our families standing dependably by to pick us up whenever we fall. For our bodies, that normal and dependable is called homeostasis.

Among the most important of the equations the body tries to balance, and one of the most neglected in terms of medical attention, is our acid-alkaline balance. The human body operates best in a neutral environment, neither very acidic nor very basic. Our bodies expend a great deal of energy and many resources maintaining this balance between the various raw materials and wastes floating throughout the body's watery environment around and within cells. Some of those components are acidic, others are alkaline, and regulatory systems are constantly at work in the digestive, excretory, and pulmonary systems to keep the balance between the two groups controlled within strict limits.

There is good cause, then to study the basics of the acid and base/alkaline concept (For our purposes, the words basic and alkaline can be used interchangeably, as they usually are. For the record, a base is also an alkali when it includes hydroxide ions (OH-). In truth, there is no single, simple answer to the question, "What are acids and bases?" There isn't even a single *complex* answer to that question. The full issue can only be explained by a number of separate, complex answers about different substances and processes with consideration given to several sometimes competing, sometimes overlapping scientific theories. However, for our purposes it is enough to think of the acid/base concept as having to do with substances that have given up electrons (H3O+ or hydronium ions) and those that have taken up electrons (OH-) from their environment. Those ions float around in solution in our cells, blood vessels, and every part of our body, giving the surrounding environment a more negative or positive charge. Because cells, proteins, and the other stuff of life function and move about differently depending on the local electrical charge of their environments, the acidic or alkaline nature of a given region of the body significantly affects its functioning.

> *Antioxidants are any compounds that prevent oxidation. In our bodies, the process of oxidation is essential to cellular respiration, the very welcome process that gives us our energy. However, there are byproducts of oxidation called free radicals, charged particles that float through the body like potential little static electrical shocks. Free radicals can trigger additional oxidation where it is unwanted (just as rusting metal is a form of oxidation), and that is where antioxidants come in. Antioxidant compounds like polyphenols and Vitamin C flow through the bloodstream as well, restoring free radicals to their harmless states and otherwise preventing them from doing their dangerous thing, which is to harm and even kill cells in our bodies.*

Frankly, the concept of acid-base homeostasis is one of the areas that are most confusing even to medical school students. Still, most of us are quite familiar with the concept of acids, which include chemicals like the hydrochloric acid that dissolves food in our stomach and the battery acid that can dissolve holes in our toys and cars. You also likely know that there are substances at the opposite end of the spectrum that have a soapy feel to them, like ammonia. You may have performed a science lab or two in your school years, combining an acid with a base to neutralize the two substances. In that lab you would have been studying the pH scale and possibly used the same litmus papers that many Earth Clinic readers now use to test their urine and other bodily fluids for levels of acidity/alkalinity.

Those litmus papers give a reading on the relative acidity or alkalinity of a liquid on the pH scale, which runs from 0 to 14 with 7 as the neutral, middle reading that is neither acidic nor basic. On the pH scale, the lower numbers are acidic, and the higher numbers increasingly basic or alkaline. Each step on the scale is a factor of 10, making a solution that reads four on the scale 10 times as acidic as a five solution and 100 times more acidic than a reading of six. What pH is actually measuring is the hydrogen ion concentration, the concentration of positively charged hydrogen ions ((H+) effectively the same as the H3O+ or hydronium ions) in a solution. More (H+) ions mean that a solution is more acidic. Since the various types of atoms in our body are constantly exchanging electrons to do their work and make their transformations, that ratio of positively to negatively charged ions that pH measures has a substantial effect on what activities can and are likely to occur in that part of the body.

In terms of the living systems that make up our bodies, scientific studies tell us that our urine should be mildly acidic, as should our saliva, at about the same pH reading of 6.4 or between 6.0 and 6.8. Our blood is healthiest when slightly alkaline, between 7.35 and 7.45. Skin is typically somewhat acidic, around a pH of 5.5, in order to fend off viruses and other pathogens that land on the skin.

LOUIS PASTEUR

While earlier cultures often thought the remarkable transition from wine to curative vinegar was likely a gift from gods and spirits, it was the French scientist Louis Pasteur who discovered the truth. Pasteur, the physicist famous for his discovery of penicillin, also was the first to determine that acetobacter bacteria converted the alcohol compounds present in cider or wine into acetic acid, the basis of vinegar.

Born the son of a French tanner in Dole, France in 1822, Louis Pasteur became a scientist working largely in physics and chemistry, eventually bringing forth innovations in many fields, although most importantly in the fields of biology and medicine.

Pasteur's contributions to human health are numerous. He opened the field of modern medicine by conclusively proving the germ theory of disease, our modern understanding that microorganisms cause many of our maladies. While the related benefits from his discovery of penicillin and subsequent antibiotics are unfathomably large, Pasteur also created the first vaccine for rabies. He created the process to eliminate pathogens in milk and other foods, a process that others came to call pasteurization in his honor.

Conversely, Pasteur found that microorganisms like the penicillin bacterium could be helpful as well, as with his discovery of the acetobacter family of bacteria that produces the wonders of the world's vinegars. Indeed, among Pasteur's major written works was Studies on Vinegar, which was published in 1868.

Of course, everything in the body is in a constant state of flux, between our own activities and the underlying metabolic processes that move materials in and out of the body. In particular, the body's respiratory and metabolic functions all produce acids as waste products, which means that the body must compensate for all that acid production by excreting acid wastes and by buffering wastes with alkaline molecules until those wastes can be excreted from the body.

In the effort to maintain acid-base homeostasis, the body's first goal is to keep the two sides facing off in even numbers of acids and bases. When that is not possible, the body uses buffers to temporarily make it as if the numbers were even. Buffering agents are substances that don't actually neutralize the pH environment. Instead, they stop acids or bases in a solution from taking up or giving off hydrogen ions (H+), effectively evening the sides by taking some of the players out of the action.

Thanks to the buffering agents and homeostatic maintenance systems that govern our acid-base balance, the body taken as a whole effectively hovers around a neutral pH of 7, and other than in our digestive system the body is unhappy and likely unhealthy if its pH in any part strays terribly far in either direction from a neutral pH. On the other hand, occasional or consistent changes in pH can be very healthy and are certainly natural. No one should be anxious about keeping exactly the same pH reading in the urine or other bodily fluid from day to day. In fact, the body will intentionally swing a pH level in one direction or another as a part of the body's defense mechanisms. A more acidic environment will kill off bacteria like those that cause strep infections and the flu, while in other cases the body seeks out a more alkaline level to combat other incipient conditions.

Before you worry overmuch about the levels of acidity and alkalinity in your body, remember we do employ a number of very strong buffering systems to constantly regulate our internal acid-base homeostasis, from simply breathing at different rates to our kidney functions. No one would recommend that you determine all of your health concerns and attempts at wellness solely on the basis of your body's overall or specific pH balances.

Nevertheless, the acid-alkaline balance was Dr. Jarvis' foremost concern, and it continues to be a prominent concern for today's naturopaths and experts in folk medicine. Often, substantial changes in the pH value of one of the body's component systems, like the blood or urine, indicate that a change in health is imminent or occurring. Such changes can indicate the body's attempt to prevent an infection from taking hold or reveal a problem in our health that is making it difficult for the body to maintain its normal homeostasis.

Surprisingly, the foods we eat have negligible effect on pH values in the body, at least taken one meal at a time. Your intensely acidic Pepsi and pickles lunch is actually going to have very little effect on the overall acidity of your body in the next several hours. After all, your gastric juices have a pH of 1.0, and the metabolic/respiratory processes that create carbon dioxide within the body simply have a far greater effect on acid concentrations than our foods could ever have. However, if your continuing diet is high in acidity and lacks the nutrients that the body needs to maintain acid-base homeostasis, then your overall diet will certainly have a significant effect on your body's overall acidity.

Consequently, adding ACV to your diet will not increase your body's overall acidity. Even if you take it regularly, the amount of ACV you consume will never be enough to make a substantial change in the acid-base balance, at least not toward the acid column. However, the potassium and other mineral components in ACV can substantially reinforce the buffering and homeostatic systems that counteract the build-up of acids in the human body. This is what makes ACV an acid that can remedy the hyper-acidity of modern diets and help the body return to acid-base homeostasis and generally more alkaline levels.

Free radicals are products of all the body's oxidation processes. They are bits of chemicals with a positive or a negative charge, which makes them very reactive in the body. This can be good - the body uses free radicals to send messages throughout the body - but these free radicals also break down the walls of our blood vessels and possibly contribute to the growth and formation of cancers.

Are You an Acid or a Base?

The alkaline/acidic balance is one thing in theory, but how does it apply to our own lives? As likely as not, you have no idea whether your body is typically alkaline or acidic. Our doctors don't ask us or tell us to monitor this fundamental part of our overall health, but it's an incredibly easy thing to check at home, and it can provide fantastic information and understanding about the state of our bodies and how they change from day to day.

Most likely you will remember running pH tests in high school chemistry class, with the testing papers that turned blue in the presence of a base and red when exposed to an acidic liquid. You can purchase these pH strips cheaply from your local drugstore. Then all you need to do is dip one strip in the stream of your urine first thing each morning to get a reading. The container for the strips will offer a color scale, and you can match it up to each morning's test strip to get a simple reading and an idea of how your body is fairing and what it needs in the day ahead.

Dr. Jarvis called urine the "first yardstick of your health." This simple morning routine of checking your urine can give you advanced warning of oncoming colds and other illnesses, alert you to sudden changes in your system, and help you to regulate your health while getting an invaluable sense of just how your body works. After all, half of being healthy is simply paying attention to your body.

In good health, urine should give a mildly acidic pH reading of around 6.4. Urine that suddenly rises to more alkaline levels is often the first sign that you are about to experience an illness, as the immune system creates a more alkaline environment to kill off pathogens in much the same way as it uses a fever to do the same. By regularly monitoring your urinary or salivary pH, you can establish a baseline for what is normal in your body, and then offer your body the dietary support it needs when those readings shift away from normal.

Apple Cider Vinegar and pH Balance

We have suggested that Apple Cider Vinegar's ability to restore alkalinity provides additional curative abilities. Go ahead and test that claim yourself. If you are going to try apple cider vinegar for allergies, or even to prevent sickness, we suggest you do an investigation of your own. Buy a pH test kit at a local pharmacy, garden nursery, or even pool supply store. You can use these kits or pH strips to test your urine to see if you are more alkaline or acid during an allergy attack, virus or bacterial infection. Once you ascertain your pH levels, you can introduce ACV into your diet, see what it does to change those pH readings, and then adjust your dosage of apple cider vinegar accordingly.

Now as we have said, the acetic acid in ACV will not measurably affect your overall acid-alkaline balance towards greater acidity. In fact, when we eat acidic foods, the pancreas secretes bicarbonate ions, which are alkaline in nature, to balance out the acidity. These alkaline ions spread throughout the body, which further helps explains the puzzle of how this acidic food can make your body more alkaline. It's yet another metabolic process your body throws into action to keep its homeostasis and maintain your proper health.

Yet beyond even that effect, the ACV tonic will add other nutrients and enzymes to your diet, help your body to draw out and make use of more of the nutrients in the foods you eat, and back up the alkalizing and normative agents in your body—all to help restore your acid-alkaline homeostasis and with that fortify your health for the long-term.

Potassium

In addition to the above ACV also contributes potassium, yet another of the critical components to acid-alkaline homeostasis, and as such it is also the other critical concept in apple cider vinegar science. In fact, the potassium we find in ACV has many roles with regard to our health and the normal functioning of our bodies.

While potassium has long been a featured listing among the vitamins and minerals on the ingredient labeling for our foods, and "check his potassium levels" has been a go-to phrase on television medical dramas, few of us actually know much about potassium. It is, in fact, an alkali metal and a reasonably common mineral. At the least, it is commonly enough available in nature that it plays a central role in all living cells, the entire kingdoms of the plants and animals included. You won't see potassium lying around on its own in nature (it reacts violently with both oxygen and water in metallic form), but it is very prevalent as an ionic salt in seawater, much like sodium, another alkali metal.

Since it is found in the cells of everything we eat, most of us get the minimum necessary supply of potassium from our diets without much effort. However, very few of us get as much potassium as we ought to, especially since a high potassium diet has been linked to a reduction in hypertension, heart disease, and stroke. Such benefits are unsurprising, as potassium plays a central role in the full spectrum of metabolic processes from the large-scale movement of our muscles to the flow of nutrients and information within the cells themselves.

Potassium's central role is probably as a component of the sodium-potassium ion pump. Chemically known as the Na+/K+-ATPase pump, the sodium-potassium pump is actually an enzyme found in the plasma membrane of all animal cells and some plant cells. It is a crucial engine for movement between the insides of our cells and the extracellular fluid. The Na+/K+-ATPase pump enzymes are found scattered numerously across the cell wall, pumping three sodium ions out of the cell and two potassium ions in with each repetition of the enzyme's functional cycle.

That sodium-potassium ion pump controls the balance of water inside of cells and the body as a whole, with potassium drawing water into the body's various cells and sodium pulling water into the blood vessels and interstitial regions of the body. The resulting ionization of the cell's interior further influences the flow of sugar, proteins, nutrients, and wastes between the intercellular and extracellular environments.

Yet the sodium-potassium pump is of even greater importance within the neurons and muscle cells, where the transfer of those positively and negatively charged ions plays a substantial role in the electrical signaling that activates those cells for movement, thought, and reaction.

Polyphenols include a wide collection of chemicals produced by plants. ACV is full of them, and they offer several benefits to human health. The tannins and flavonoids in ACV are subsets of the polyphenol class. Similar polyphenols can be found in most plant life, but they are particularly abundant in berries, nuts, chocolate, olives, grapes, and beverages such as beer, wine, and tea. Medical studies continue to test polyphenols as antioxidants that might comb the body for free radicals, thereby reducing the threats of cancer and cardiovascular disease.

Despite the extensive need for potassium in all these processes and regulatory systems of the body, our Earth Clinic readers are often most concerned with potassium in its role as a fairly strong alkalizing agent, counteracting the body's acid-making metabolic processes. The very flow of nutrients, wastes, and materials that potassium makes possible itself plays a substantial role in maintaining acid-base homeostasis within each cell. It does so simply by making the continual flow of alkaline and acid molecules possible within and without the cell walls. That flow allows the cell to find and maintain its acid-base balance. In particular, the acidic wastes of each cell's metabolic processes require the electrical potential energy that the sodium-potassium pump maintains in order to power other metabolic pumps that move waste out of the cell.

In addition to the flow of life that potassium fuels, as an alkali metal potassium is itself a strongly alkalizing agent. Compounds like potassium citrate are sometimes even recommended as alkalizing supplements or antacids. Actually, potassium citrate (as you would find in citrus fruits) acts as a much stronger alkalizing agent within the body than the typical sodium bicarbonate, thanks to the efficacy of potassium. Fortunately for us, all we need is a little ACV.

If you are a farmer or gardener, this central role played by potassium is no doubt less foreign for you than for the rest of us. Potassium (K) has always been a part of the typical NPK fertilizer mixture of nitrogen, phosphorus, and potassium that includes the primary nutrients plants need for complete health. Without potassium, plants yellow, whither, and die with the results particularly visible in their leaves.

Of course, human beings don't exactly wilt. Yet the inversion our diets have undergone – suddenly including far more salt and therefore sodium than potassium, when the ratio should be entirely reversed – has caused many of us to likewise experience side effects from potassium shortages. For us, yellow and wilting is equal to continuing fatigue, general symptoms of depression, muscle weakness, poor reflexes, and heart irregularities. All are symptoms of a low potassium supply in the human body, and not surprisingly those symptoms often show up in conditions for which ACV provides relief.

In general, it is not necessary to aggressively supplement your diet with potassium. The modest increases in potassium that we can get from regular use of the ACV tonic or from foods like potatoes and bananas can provide the improvement we need. However, if you do take a potassium supplement or make extensive use of ACV you should rest easy in knowing that unless you have a kidney condition, it is more or less impossible to get too much potassium from your diet.

Flavonoids, which are sometimes also called bioflavonoids, are antioxidant molecules created by and reasonably common in plants, although some plants and plant-products offer significantly more flavonoids than others. Green and black teas, dark chocolate, and red wine are among the foods that have popped up in the news as cancer-fighters and protectors of the cardiovascular system, thanks to their flavonoid content. In addition to combating and preventing cancers, flavonoids have been found to reduce allergic reactions and inflammation.

The Supporting Cast

While ACV's supply of potassium and its dual acid and alkaline effects are often the central components of the ACV health benefits we enjoy, the wide variety of conditions ACV addresses and the success with which it addresses any health condition owe much to the large team of components you find in organic ACV.

We have made some mention of the phytochemicals in ACV, which is simply to say chemicals made by plants. Most of them are unstudied, but where some research has been done we find that they are astonishingly productive of continuing health even in the smallest quantities. Unpasteurized ACV offers a host of cancer-fighting antioxidants, metabolism-revving enzymes, and nutrient-releasing probiotics.

Soluble fiber, specifically pectin, also provides substantial benefit from within the ACV tonic. Soluble fiber is a phrase that rolls off the seemingly knowledgeable tongues of many a commercial actor, but with very little explanation as to why it might be so important. Soluble and insoluble fiber are the two types of plant-derived dietary fibers. Insoluble fiber absorbs water and passes through the digestive system unchanged, sweeping up garbage along the way. Whereas soluble fiber is fermented in the digestive tract, transformed thereby into materials that promote digestion and overall health, according to continuing scientific findings. Yet pectin's most effective trick as a soluble fiber seems to be in binding with cholesterol to carry it safely out of the body.

Pectin should be somewhat familiar to those who have made jams and jellies, or who eagerly watched their grandmothers do the same. It is sold as a gelling agent that turns raw fruit juices into jellied forms. Pectin is the natural product of many plants, is often found in cell walls, and as a part of our diets it is an important soluble fiber. It doesn't offer much nutrition, but pectin is a tremendous aid to health in the way that it binds with and speeds the passing of cholesterol out of the digestive tract, reducing blood cholesterol levels and the threat of atherosclerosis.

The soluble fiber pectin that is found in ACV plays several roles, as we have highlighted them. In the vascular system it helps control the use and presence of simple sugars, helping to relieve some of the burden from insulin. When it reaches the intestines, pectin also is broken down into simpler substances that aid in complete digestion of the other food in our guts.

Kaempferol and quercetin may be two of the most beneficial of the flavonoids, and both are found in abundance in apples and apple cider vinegar. Researchers at UCLA's Johnson Cancer Center found that these flavonoids, among others, were effective in reducing the incidence of lung cancer and seemed to help in stopping and killing cancerous cell growth.

With its antioxidants, ACV is again addressing the critical issue of ions running free and unbalanced throughout our bodies. Those ions are necessary for many biological processes that are essential to life, but like unbridled teenagers those ions will "oxidize" other substances in the body wherever they find them, activating biological processes simply because they can, though such uncontrolled reactions lead to such things as cardiovascular damage and cancer.

And that in a nutshell is the basic role of ACV in the body: shutting down unwanted processes and imbalances on the one hand while on the other hand activating desirable systems in the body that need a little boost to get going. In the end, that is what the science of apple cider vinegar comes down to—reestablishing balance, homeostasis of all kinds and in every part of the body. Just ask your yoga instructor, your football coach, or your mentor about the value of that kind of support. They'll tell you that when we have balance, we can handle anything that comes at us.

Chapter 4

IT'S GOOD FOR THAT TOO: AILMENTS REMEDIED BY ACV

Now down to the nitty-gritty. Let's talk about what Apple Cider Vinegar might do for you and your family.

Despite the remarkable number of conditions apple cider vinegar has been found to address, the common recommendation for treatment with ACV is as consistent and simple as taking a medication three times a day — or drinking a glass of water. Beginning with Dr. Jarvis, the sort of godfather of modern ACV therapy, the standard dosage has been to slowly drink the following "ACV Tonic":

ACV Tonic

- *2 teaspoons organic, unpasteurized ACV*
- *8 oz of water*
- *Sweetener to taste (honey and genuine maple syrup are best)*

After a decade of experience and reader feedback on the Earth Clinic website, we now recommend that our readers raise the water-to-ACV ratio as a way to reduce the minimal side effects of steady acid consumption. Unless you have a low acid condition or are looking for the antibiotic effects of the acid itself, a more diluted/lower acidity mixture will prevent any possible damage to tooth enamel, the throat, or a sudden change in the body's homeostasis (for further discussion of possible ACV side effects, see our section in chapter 5).

In the case of conditions where you are using the acidity itself to treat an ailment — for conditions like acid reflux, sore throats, expectorant cough, and bronchitis — we recommend from 2 teaspoons up to 2 tablespoons of ACV in 8 ounces of water. Standard ACV acidity levels, which will be around 5% in any bottle of vinegar, have been proven strong enough to kill off many viruses, bacteria, and fungi. Concentrations as low as 1% are still effective and about the right dilution for prophylactic treatment, as with a skin wash or a treatment compress. Internal treatments, such as douching for a vaginal infection or catheterization, can be accomplished with acetic acid concentrations of 0.25-1% acidity, that is a ratio of water to ACV of 5:1 or greater.

For many people, their preferred internal dosage is best taken three times a day, either before or with each meal. With the diluted mixture, you will likely find yourself slowly sipping the tonic throughout the day, which is the best way to keep your body in a constantly alkalized state and slowly absorbing the nutrients ACV provides. You will also likely find that it helps to maintain a more constant energy level throughout your day.

A more diluted ACV drink may also make it unnecessary to add any sweetener. Dr. Jarvis and many others have promoted honey and to a lesser extent maple syrup for the legitimate additional health benefits of those sweeteners; however, at this time most of us are rightfully more concerned about weight issues, and so it is best to reduce additional calorie sources wherever we can. Therefore, our new recommendation for drinking the ACV tonic is the following:

- *2 teaspoons organic apple cider vinegar*
- *8-20 ounces water*
- *Mix and sip throughout the day*

However, you should feel free to add a natural sweetener if you feel the need. In fact, many of our readers experiment with adding ACV to apple cider, apple juice, tomato juice, herbal teas, and any number of other liquids. You could likewise add a couple of teaspoons of ACV to your salad with much the same effect.

Apple cider vinegar is also excellent for use as an external treatment, as an antiseptic wash for the skin as well as in the form of a compress to alleviate skin and subcutaneous conditions, but we will address those other possibilities as we present suggestions alongside reader feedback on each of the conditions to follow.

All of the feedback in the coming sections was pulled from the Earth Clinic site within a short period between September 2009 and June 2010, as a small representation of typical feedback about ACV remedies. The feedback you are about to read can still be found on the site.

Without further ado, here are the top cures from ACV treatment, according to the experiences of our online community:

Acid Reflux

Acid reflux, sometimes referred to as GERD (gastroesophageal reflux disease), has become simultaneously a tremendous health issue and a huge market for pharmaceutical companies. However, Earth Clinic readers have found long-term relief with simple ACV treatment. Acid reflux is a problem of the digestive system characterized by intense heartburn-like pain from food and stomach acids that return up the esophageal track. The pain can disturb a sufferer's sleep, reduce nutrient intake, and utterly disrupt life, as Angie from North Dakota found:

> "I have been having a problem with reflux for several years now. I had been on prescription meds, but after seeing side effects others had listed online, I never stayed on them very long. I was also having severe anxiety problems where I felt like I couldn't breathe,

> felt nauseated, hot and all at very random times. I had tried ACV once before with terrible results. Earlier this week, I had the worst reflux burning I'd ever had and was about to succumb to the "purple pill" once again. I got on this site and read all the testimonials on ACV and decided that with how bad I was feeling, I might as well give it a try once again. I didn't have the organic kind with "the mother", so I just tried the regular. In about an hour, I realized that I didn't have ANY burning, pain or the sensation of anything coming back up. I slept like a baby and without keeping a cough drop in my cheek for the first time in… waaaay too long… years, probably. I have been using it for three days now and I cannot believe what a difference it has made! I didn't realize how disruptive my reflux was! I have not had any of those old anxiety feelings whatsoever since ACV! I believe it was all connected to the reflux […] I will continue the ACV and spread the word! Thanks to this site and to all who have put their testimonials on here. I never would have tried it if it weren't for you!"

Readers have been in favor of the ACV treatment for Acid Reflux at a rate of 15 to 1 (Yea to Nay) in their responses. Those with the best response probably experience GERD or reflux due to too little acid production by their own bodies. Too much acid is also a possibility with these conditions, but whether more people suffer from too much or too little acid is uncertain and people with both levels seem to benefit from ACV, as you will see here:

> **Ted from Bennington, Vermont:** "I also have suffered from acid reflux for about a year. Took acid-dissolving tablets, which only temporarily alleviated the symptoms. Discovered ACV on this site and after taking two doses (2 tsp. of ACV in 8 oz. of water) in one day, I felt better for the next five days than I had for months. Problem totally gone. While looking for information about ACV, I discovered at least one site that purported to pop the ACV balloon by declaring ACV has no medicinal or health-giving properties, etc. Amusing to see that the site's sponsors were all pharmaceutical and health care/insurance companies. Gee, how about that! As if those folks would tell the truth if their lives depended on it."

Cajun from Opelousas, Louisiana: "For most of my young adolescent life, I lived virtually every day of my life with acid reflux; baking soda when convenient, antacid tablets during other times. Once computers came into the Engineering profession, I daily combined about 3-4 oz of ACV with ice and water as my [32oz] drink. I've been without acid reflux for so long now (~35 years) that I have forgotten how long it took to relieve/cure my acid reflux. I'll be 70yo in 4 months and I never have any relapses. YES, ACV does 'cure' acid reflux."

D from Pittsburgh, Pennsylvania: "I took the purple pill for years and years until it stopped working. I went to the doc for coughing fits, and hoarseness not realizing it was connected to acid reflux. He doubled my prescription of the purple pill to 2 a day, nothing got better in fact I got worse. I started searching for a natural remedy, found this website and tried the apple cider vinegar plus honey and water. It started working immediately to fix the acid reflux. I went off the purple pill immediately and stayed on the ACV plus honey. It took 2-3 months but my hoarseness went away and eventually the cough."

Bud from Benton, Arkansas: "Apple cider vinegar and honey has definitely helped my acid reflux problem. I took a 2 liter (2 qt) plastic bottle, which is 8- 8oz servings and added 8oz ACV and 4oz of honey and filled with H2O. I started 6 days ago and drink 2 8oz glasses a day, one before breakfast and one before dinner. It has worked wonders! No more coughing and regurgitating at night and the lump in my throat is about gone. On day 4, I decided to skip the one before dinner, just to see if it made a difference and I was coughing and food was coming up in the night. I went to the kitchen and drank a glass and slept the rest of the night without a problem. Before I started this, I would spray my throat several times a night to try and keep from coughing. I haven't sprayed my throat one time since I started doing this. I would recommend trying it to anyone. It may not work for everyone, but, so far it has worked great for me with no side effects!"

As a general treatment for Acid Reflux conditions, we recommend up to 2 Tablespoons of ACV with 8oz water, drunk before and with your meal to prepare your stomach for food.

Acne

Acne is everyone's problem at one point or another, but as it is primarily a problem of too much oil production and then contamination by bacteria, ACV is great for treating it. The acid in an ACV wash (dab a cotton pad in a bit of ACV, then wipe the face) will kill the bacteria and dissolve and wash away excess oils, leaving your skin clear and shining. Just be careful not to get too much sun after washing with ACV, as it will sensitize you a bit to UV rays. You might also want to remember that dabbing yourself with the light scent of salad dressing isn't going to be the best choice for a first date!

Additionally enjoying the ACV drink once or twice a day will give your body the nutrients and hydration it needs to be acne-free.

Hippiechick from Laurel, Maryland: "ACV has nearly cured my acne. I have had acne since my 1st menstrual cycle in 6th grade. I'm 35-years old now. I have tried everything you can think of... the only thing that has worked is Raw Organic Apple Cider Vinegar."

Elaine from Pueblo, Colorado: "I'm 26 and have never had problems with Acne until about 6 months ago. I broke out on my cheeks and my chest. I have tried everything and even went to the dermatologist. He prescribed me Retin-a and an antibacterial face wash. Neither has helped at all. A couple weeks ago I read about ACV on this site and started using it every morning and night on my face. I wash my face with an organic face wash, then use a cotton ball to apply ACV to my face. I let it dry for about 5-6 minutes then I apply a moisturizer. Make sure to moisturize afterwards or it will really dry your skin. I also have been drinking a splash of ACV mixed with water daily. I can't believe how good my skin looks. The acne is almost completely gone, replaced by a healthy glow. I would recommend this to anyone with acne problems. It really is amazing."

Holly from Portland, Oregon: "Apple Cider Vinegar CURED my non-inflammatory acne MUCH MUCH better than Retin-A!! I have a prescription for Retin-A, and have been taking it for months. It smells and I know it's bad for your skin as far as sun damage goes, so I've never used it on my face, where for the last few years, I've had small under the skin bumps that are sort of annoying. I thought others were exaggerating on overnight success but I kid you not, I dipped a cotton swab in ACV and ran it over the area, went to bed, woke up excited to see the results, ran my fingers over it—baby bottom smooth! Incredible!"

Radha from Urbandale, Iowa: "Pure apple cider vinegar cured my acne in a week and a half. I have normal skin but tend to get the usual breakout around the end of the month. At one point, my entire left cheek was covered in hard, red, itchy pimples and clear little dots everywhere. I started using a gentle exfoliator for my face wash. Then I would dip a cotton ball in ACV and rub it all over my face. Just a thin layer will do. Then I would sit for a little bit and let it dry. The smell is something you'll get used to but the first night is terrible. Have the thin layer of ACV dry then apply just a light moisturizer then go to sleep. Make sure all your pimples and such are covered by the ACV. You aren't going to get amazing results over night if you have severe acne; but after about 3-4 days you'll start to see them slowly dry up. If you start to see puss rise up in some LEAVE THEM ALONE. Picking them will only leave a scar. This is my daily routine, my face has cleared so amazingly. "

Allergies

It's not clear that ACV should have any direct effect on allergy symptoms, but our readers have reported very positive results in some cases, which may be the result of ACV's ability to strengthen the body and the immune system in general. In the case of allergies, adding locally produced, unfiltered honey to your ACV dose may be the best choice. Honey taken just before the onset of allergy season can prime the body to effectively ignore seasonal allergens.

Charley from Pinellas Park, Florida: "Due to possible pollen allergy, I suffered stuffy nose and chest congestion since early January of this year until this month of April. Two days ago, I surfed this site looking for relief and was inspired by so many testimonials about apple cider vinegar. I mixed 2 tablespoons each of apple cider vinegar and honey plus a dash of cayenne powder. In a mug I heated the mixture with water for 3 minutes and drank it. Just after few minutes I realized that this is a miracle drink, and for two nights I have had good sleep and my condition has improved by 75%."

Chris from Auburn, Alabama: "First off, this is the most amazing site I've ever come across. I've had acute allergies for 10 years now. For the first 5 years, I just dealt with it, but as I've gotten older, it's gotten worse. I usually end up bed ridden with sinusitis, fever, terrible headaches, etc. before all is better. The last 5 years, I have taken an antibiotic virtually every time I had an outbreak (about every 2 months), and everyone knows how bad that is for our bodies. Since I found the ACV cure a year ago, I've had ONE outbreak. I cured both of my last outbreaks without antibiotics in a matter of 3 or 4 days. I now drink ACV daily."

Arthritis

The symptoms of arthritis and the progression of pain and disfiguration are largely a result of deficiencies in mineral uptake, circulation of bodily fluids, and immune system regulation. All of these factors can be improved by ACV treatment, which improves nutrient absorption, circulatory system function, and homeostasis throughout the body. ACV can also help dissolve the calcium deposits that play into arthritis symptoms.

Larry from Bartlett, Illinois: "Been into holistic health for a few years now and stumbled upon Earth Clinic a few months ago [...] I broke my left elbow about 22 years ago in a motorcycle accident and the Dr. then told me it would give me trouble later in life. He was completely correct, as over the past 1-1/2 years it has gone from a noticeable throb to outright excruciating PAIN! Some mornings I couldn't even extend it fully and certainly could not do anything physically stressful. After reading about ACV and arthritis I began using it as directed with about two tablespoons in water, sipping it throughout the day. Within 10 minutes of the first sips the pain subsided. I'm now into the fourth day and I'm a new man."

Peter from Manila, Philippines: "I am presently reading the book "Arthritis And Folk Medicine " written by D.C. Jarvis. M.D. [....] To explain how [ACV] works in arthritis, he uses the analogy of the tea kettle with the calcium build up, which when boiled with ACV solution, the calcium deposit is dissolved. So it is this ability to precipitate "dead" calcium that is his explanation as to how it works with arthritis.

What caught my attention was the case of the ACV fed calf that was dehorned at ten months of age and was found to have full calcium horns whereas others unfed with ACV were hollow. That seems to show that it helps the fuller utilization of calcium. Another example is the calves supplemented with ACV being bigger boned and bodied than the unsupplemented ones.

> Another example was that the butcher paid a higher price for dairy cows that were "vinegared" because the meat was more tender than that of others. This is interesting because it shows a good circulation throughout the animal not only indicating no arthritis but also no rheumatism - the hardening of the muscle tissues [....] So how does acv work in eliminating arthritis? Dr Jarvis's answer would be that it assists calcium metabolism and rids the body of badly utilized calcium that causes calcium buildups, which is the cause of arthritic pain, and when the excess calcium goes, so does the pain."

Arthritis sufferers might also benefit from a topical application of ACV, in addition to drinking it.

- *Combine 1/4 cup of ACV with 1 1/2 cups of hot (but not scalding) water, and soak the affected body part in this mixture.*
- *For areas too large to soak directly, try soaking a cloth in an ACV mixture of the above ratio and putting it on the affected area. Wrap a towel over the wet cloth to keep in the heat. Keep the wrap on for ten minutes, then remove.*
- *You can repeat treatment after the joint has cooled for ten minutes.*

Athlete's Foot

The fungus that causes athlete's foot can be killed with a topical solution of ACV or with a foot bath, as Marian from Tasmania, Australia has found:

"Hi all, I read on your site (I think) that bathing feet in cider vinegar for a minimum of 6 weeks would cure athletes foot. I have had this condition since a teenager, I'm now 58. Usually didn't notice it too much in winter when I was wearing shoes but each summer my heels would crack and give me grief. So I was constantly putting healing cream on with band-aids and this went on all summer. This year it started in the winter, and I noticed that my feet were peeling also. So I quite religiously rubbed organic cider vinegar on my feet each night, and dried them off in front of the fire, an evening ritual before bed. My feet are now completely clear of peeling and splitting and feel so good."

Bacterial Vaginosis

The antibacterial properties of acetic acid can be put to good use against conditions like bacterial vaginosis, without the side effects of antibiotic treatment.

Sake from New York, New York: "Apple Cider Vinegar. I am a believer: I had recurrent B.V for almost 1 year. Went to the doctor twice, got 2 courses of metrodinazole. That worked for a while but B.V kept coming back until just this past Saturday, I was lurking right here on Earth Clinic and decided to buy some at the health food store. I swear the B.V cleared up that SAME DAY. It's been 2 days now, and nary an itch!"

KH from Oklahoma City, Oklahoma: "I have used regular vinegar for years now to clear up any problems in the region. I just buy the disposable douche bottles in the box with solution already in them, pour the solution out and replace with 1 part vinegar and 2 parts water. Do this twice a day for 2 days and then I'm fine. It does sting a little at first, but nothing unbearable. The vinegar odor does not last long at all (maybe an hour or two). ACV is alot more powerful than regular vinegar so I would imagine it works better."

Bladder Infection/Bladder Issues

Acetic acid in ACV works together with the vinegar's natural ability to boost and regulate the immune system to help restore order to your bladder and urinary tract. Many readers have reported great success in using the ACV tonic to cure urinary tract infections (UTI) in particular.

Katrina from St. Louis, Missouri: "I had the worst UTI I've ever had. I was in so much pain I could not think or focus on anything else. I took a swig of ACV WITH WATER and in less than twenty minutes the pain was tolerable. Then I put some in a water bottle and sipped on it for a day. I felt completely better. That kind of pain can bring a person to tears. I don't have insurance and I am sooooo happy I found this site. Thank You, Thank You, Thank You!"

Elizabeth from New York, New York: "I was having another episode with my recurring urinary tract infection and I remembered my co-worker informing me that her sister drinks ACV and swears by it. So, I had my husband go and buy me a bottle. I boiled a cup of water and 2 tsp of ACV. I could not believe it half way through I started feeling immediate relief."

Milly from Wales, United Kingdom: "Urinary Problems: Started taking apple cider vinegar after reading of all the health benefits. I really like it with tomato juice. After about a week I noticed that I sleep through the night without needing to get up to visit the bathroom. I am very happy about this and feel far more energetic during the day."

Blood Pressure

The ACV tonic seems to have a dramatic and almost immediate effect on high blood pressure and hypertension. Our readers simply report their positive results with pleasure, but the medical theory is that ACV relaxes the cell walls of the veins and arteries while clearing out deposits on the interior walls of the vascular system, allowing for easier blood flow and therefore less pressure.

Murali from San Jose, California: "As someone who has had essential hypertension for many years (160mm/100mm, unmedicated and 130/90 with three medicines - angiotensin blocker, Ca channel blocker, and beta blocker), I have been on the quest for a drug free cure. I am 47, in good health, work out every day (ran a marathon last year), and watch what I eat carefully. The doctors have not been able to ID what is the cause of my rampant high BP.

I have begun the ACV protocol and I am noticing substantial improvement over the last few weeks. But more importantly, several studies have been done in Japan (medically accepted double blind studies). Please note that in Japan, vinegar is a part of the food (sushi has vinegar/rice)[....] The key is to look for the impact of acetic acid on hypertension. Acetic acid is the primary component of ACV. Acetic acid has a substantial and sustained impact on high BP AFTER SEVERAL WEEKS."

Lauren910 from Orlando, Florida: "I am 28 years old and have had pre-hypertension for about the last year... usual readings were anywhere from 120-130/80-87. I stumbled upon this site in hopes for a natural remedy to lower my numbers. I was giving the raw, unfiltered ACV to my pets (just a bit in their water) and I had never tried it myself. For days 1 & 2 I used 2 tbsp. 3 times a day diluted in 10 ounces of water, then went to 2 tsp. 3 times a day.

All I have to say is that the results for me were amazing. After 4 days of taking ACV, my numbers are already lower. I just took my BP this morning and it was 110/63, and this is the average since I've been taking ACV. My fiance and I work in the medical industry and have a very expensive, trusted digital BP cuff we use here at home, so I am not worried about these results not being accurate."

Celteyes from Pearland, Texas writes: "I was diagnosed with exercise induced hypertension about a month ago. I am very lucky as the cardiologist told me he believes in natural medicine and he gave me until February to get better before he would put me on blood pressure meds. The apple cider vinegar has worked. I love it so much I drink it at least 3 times daily. I put 1 tablespoon in about 8 oz. water. I add 3 packet of real lemon and 2 packets of truvia. I add ice and it tastes like a tangy lemonade.

Initially when I was worked up they had to stop the treadmill because I went in with normal BP and in 2 minutes it was 220/118. I was shocked. Never in my life have I had this problem. Last week I was running many errands and walked back and forth across Target twice. I felt so tired I thought uh oh I better check my B/P. I went to the pharmacy and it read 130/80. That is still not my usual low BP but I think that is great after running around all day"

Lori from Laurel, Mississippi: "My blood pressure had gotten to be in the high 140/100 give or take a few fluctuating points daily. I read your site because I didn't want to be put on medication. I wanted to try an alternative route to lower my blood pressure. I tried apple cider vinegar (regular type from grocery) and no change. I purchased a natural ACV with the mother and my blood pressure was lower within days of using this. I drink 2tsp in a glass of water about 3x per day. It has also curbed my appetite for sweets and other junk foods. I have lost about 20 pounds in less than 3 months doing this."

Burns and Sunburns

Pour, soak, or dab ACV over a burned patch of skin immediately after being burned to clean and soothe the inflamed area. The pain should almost immediately ease, and readers further report that after treatment there will be much less pain than would be expected, quick healing, and significantly reduced scarring. ACV is best used for immediate first aid treatment on burns only, as the acetic acid may only inflame the healing skin with later treatment.

Bursitis

The swelling of the bursa sacs around our joints can cause intense pain, but ACV provides needed minerals while fostering better circulation of liquids and nutrients between cell walls and the circulatory system. Try both the ACV tonic and a direct ACV-soaked wrap or 5:1 water and ACV soak.

> **Stephen from Birzebbugia, Malta:** "Bursitis cured with ACV. I am over 50 and had a bad fall, landed on my elbow. It swelled and I thought it would go away, it didn't. Three months after I started putting ACV on it, and it remained the same. Then I soaked a piece of cloth in ACV, kept it on the swelling with an elbow support sleeve, almost day & night, and after one day it went down by 15%. I also was careful not to hit it again. On 2nd and 3rd day, down by 75%. That ugly swelling has gone and I am hoping for complete healing."

Canker Sores

Treat canker sores with a cotton swab dipped in ACV or an ACV gargle. Be aware that there will be pain, but you should find quick relief and remission thereafter. Be cautious: some readers report that ACV treatment can actually increase the number of canker sores, and this seems to depend on the sort of mouth lesions you suffer from.

> **Victoria from Gold Coast, Australia:** "I cured two nasty painful mouth ulcers which I'd had for a week using the ACV remedy on the website. I just soaked a cotton tip in it and held it on the ulcers for 10 minutes. It did burn a lot at first, but then it just felt numb. The next day I woke up and it felt much better. I applied it again that day, and they have now disappeared.
>
> I was taking a Vitamin C supplement at the time which was of 'orange color' as well, which I think is what caused the ulcers in the first place!"

> **Gloria from Santa Rosa, California:** "I recently had an awful canker sore and it was 4am and couldn't sleep because the pain bothered me. I remembered reading on Earth Clinic about a canker sore remedy, but I couldn't remember if it was with ACV or Cayenne pepper (both are my go to ingredients when I'm sick/sore throat) so I decided to use both! I dipped a Q-tip in ACV then sprinkled cayenne pepper on it and applied it directly to the canker sore. It stung at first, but the cayenne helped relieve the pain, and both seemed to help the sore tremendously! I woke up, and the pain was gone and it is now evening and I forgot I even had it!"

Cold and Flu

While it's still not that long awaited cure for the common cold or a perfect safeguard against the flu, regular ACV tonics can strengthen the immune system and keep the body properly balanced between those acidic and alkaline states that will help kill off viral invaders. Once infected, ACV can relieve your symptoms and offer the nutrients necessary to speed you back to health.

Great Tip: To clear your breathing passageways, cut out a hand-sized square from a paper bag and soak that paper in ACV. Then place the paper over your chest, directly on the skin, and breathe deeply for about 20 minutes. You should experience extended relief and find that the mucus in your chest is breaking up.

Shabbycrafter from Dos Palos, California: "For the past two days my daughter has had a horribly sore throat with white spots on it. She's had a fever, body aches, and sniffles as well. After calling around and finding that the local doctors were booked up and the rural clinic would be $250 just to see the doctor, I decided to figure out how to help her myself. I remembered a friend suggesting ACV so I gave it a try. I gave my daughter (18 years old) 2 tablespoons of ACV in an 8 oz. glass of water. She sat and sipped on it for a while. Her sore throat immediately calmed to the point where she was able to fall asleep and slept most of the night. Around 6:30 am she woke up and did the same routine again and is up and around today looking better than she has in days. I should add here that along with the ACV I gave her an over-the-counter pain reliever as well. From now on, I've decided I'm going to treat everything I can in this manner. The treatment worked better than anything I've ever seen! Amazing!"

Patti from Aston, Pennsylvania: "I became ill with upper respiratory symptoms on Wednesday, and by Friday morning I was unable to go to work. On Saturday, I was so congested I could not breathe out of my nose. The over the counter medication had stopped working and by nightfall, I knew I was in trouble and would not be able to sleep. Suffering from an unbearable headache, overall aches and pains with fever, in desperation [...] I came across your website and sent my husband to the store to buy the ACV. I took 2 T in 8 oz of warm water for my first dose at midnight and woke up at 4am and realized I could breathe - my nose had cleared! I took another dose before going to sleep, and another around noon. I felt reasonably well to cook dinner on Monday night and went back to work on Tuesday. This remedy is nothing short of a miracle for me and I cannot wait to share it with friends and family. Now that I feel better, I am anxious to investigate the rest of your site. ACV will definitely be a regular part of my diet, as I am a chronic sinus sufferer. Antibiotics offer some relief, but do not cure the problem. I thank you from the bottom of my heart for posting this natural remedy."

Marixpress from Bronx, New York: "At the first sign of flu or cold, I drank 2 tablespoons of organic ACV with about 8oz of warm water, a squeeze of lemon & honey for taste, every morning for about 3 days. Almost everyone in the household is sick, however, the ones that tried this concoction never did get sick. Thank you to Earth Clinic for this wonderful recipe!!"

Cured!!! from Woodstock, Georgia: "Yea, for ACV!!! Thank God for this site! I did a frantic search after my husband and I were both attacked by a wicked flu bug that has lasted almost 3 weeks. We're finally over the worst symptoms; but the cough (especially his) was the very last thing to go... and it wasn't going without a fight. For 2 weeks, we had tried "everything" including OTC drugs. I also had severe phlegm in the back of my throat, and had lots of nasal mucous. Both were extremely difficult to expel; and his cough was so consistent that it caused him headaches and stomach cramping. I tried the solution of 4 tbspns OJ, 2 tbspns honey and 2 tbspns ACV... within 1 hour we were both relieved of the symptoms and before the day was over, we knew we were on to the cure! We heated our recipe to make it a little easier to digest. It doesn't taste too bad, but its a long way from tasting good, and the strong taste is "oh, so worth it!"

Cold Sores

Herpes-related cold sores can be a recurring frustration, but topical treatment with an ACV wash can reduce their duration and perhaps keep them from reappearing as often.

Pundon2010 from Charlotte, North Carolina: "On this past Monday I started to have that "tingling" feeling on my lip meaning the beginning of a cold sore breakout. By mid afternoon I was right, a huge blister in the corner of my mouth ouch! After reading the numerous reviews on ACV as a cold sore remedy, I decided to give it a try. On this past Tuesday I went to the store and got the ACV and put some on a cotton ball. Without a moment's notice the cold sore started to burn like someone had thrown perm on my face! But after a few moments the burning sensation went away. About an hour later the cold sore had reduced in size. I did the same thing again before I went to bed. When I woke up the next morning the cold sore had reduced in size about 1/2 inch and had began to crack as if it was drying out already!! YAY!! I thought, but to my dismay there was yet another cold sore peeking its ugly head out from beneath my lower lip. After having success with the other sore, I kept reapplying the ACV with a cotton ball 4-5 times a day for both sores for approximately 3 days. Today is Friday and I am glad to say that both sores are gone!"

Cough

Irritation, infection, and accumulations of phlegm can all be relieved by the acidic and antibacterial/antiviral properties of ACV. A warm ACV tonic will be particularly effective, and the addition of honey will help to soothe your throat while treating it.

Adriana from Sofia, Bulgaria: "I did not see any postings on ACV's ability to cure cough. It works as a cough syrup. I had terrible cough and flu this winter. So I searched online and found out that equal amounts of ACV and honey in a cup of water work miracles. I tried it and felt instant relief. It has anti-viral properties and helps fight the flu.

Here in Bulgaria it is also traditionally used to lower fever. The way it's done is to wet a cloth with the vinegar and cover the forehead and temples. The vinegar and the cooling effect of the wet cloth work together."

Tivins from Queensland, Australia: "I caught a bad cold recently, while the medicine from the chemist stops the cold, I can't stop the cough that came after it. The cough was very bad. Feels like there's something ticklish on my throat and makes me wanna cough it out but I can't. At night, I'm not able to sleep, just cough and cough till I got cramps in the stomach. I looked for the cure in this site. (I save this site on my desktop). I took 3 capfuls of apple cider vinegar with my normal morning tea with either sugar or honey with warm water. In a couple of hours, my coughs lessened and the sore I felt in my throat from coughing felt better. My runny nose also stops and I feel so much better. Thank you Earth Clinic, you make my day!"

Dandruff

The cause of many skin conditions comes back to an imbalance in the skin's naturally acidic state, and an ACV wash can help to remedy that shortcoming in the case of dandruff as with other skin conditions while also improving the skin's ability to circulate nutrients and moisture within the body. Many shampoos can be rather alkaline, disrupting your scalp's normal condition, and an ACV wash can counteract that imbalance.

Maya2141 from Cambridge, Massachusetts: "I have been suffering from Seborrhea for most of my adult life and used all possible medicated and non-medicated shampoos, nothing seemed to help. The only thing that worked was steroid creams, and after I stopped them, it came back. I turned to the internet and found the ACV cure on EC. I have used it religiously for two weeks and it's working.

I read another user's remark and got myself a color applicator from a beauty store and poured half ACV and half water. I apply it everyday after shampooing, rub it into the scalp and leave it for 2 to 5 minutes. It stinks like vinegar when the hair is wet, but once dry, no smell. There is no to minimal scaling and absolutely no itching in the hair. Since it's only a couple of weeks, I am going it give it more time to completely get rid of the scaling. Note: I use an organic shampoo, with all natural ingredients and no sulfates. And since using ACV, I have skipped using the conditioner, the ACV leaves hair soft, shiny and detangled."

Ascha4 from Springfield, Illinois: "I didn't suffer from severe dandruff or have any scalp conditions but just had bad, very visible dandruff in my brunette hair. I used one application of half ACV and half water, and was cured. I also switched to shampoo without any sulfates in it, that helps too for maintenance."

Dermatitis

Acute inflammations of the skin can be red, irritating, itchy, and painful. An ACV wash and a continued ACV tonic habit can restore your skin to its normal, weakly acidic state (pH 5.5) to protect against pathogens and toxins that can irritate the skin, resulting in dermatitis.

Clare from London, United Kingdom: "I have had what seems to be perioral dermatitis for nearly 20 years, have tried all sorts [of treatments] to manage this but for the past week have used ACV in water... very quickly cleared up and very very grateful to this site. It gradually started to reappear when I went a day without sipping the ACV and am anxious about taking this long term but so pleased that I seem to be heading in the right direction :-)"

Tracey from Calgary, Alberta, Canada: "I must begin by expressing a sentiment I have read many times throughout this site yet feel compelled to reiterate just the same. I am simply agog at the time, money and heartache - especially the heartache - I wouldn't have had to spend if just one of my doctors had known of the effective, natural cures I have found here at Earth Clinic [....] After almost two months of being mostly trapped indoors with perioral dermatitis, I found this site. For five days I followed this regime:

• 2 tbsp of pure organic apple cider vinegar in 16oz of water, 2-3x/day
• Saturation of a cotton pad application of straight apple cider vinegar to the affected area 2-3x/day

Less than a week later, 85% of the hideously shaming rash had cleared. Rather than a solid mass of red bumps (scattered with whiteheads) from nose to chin, the condition appeared as individual spots, more like regular acne. I noticed these spots were stubborn and seemed somewhat resistant to the ACV. Additionally, in areas that had healed, hyper-pigmentation was extensive.

I searched about this last issue and found the page re: hydrogen peroxide and acne. Yesterday (day 6), I did this three times:
• Dip cotton swab [...] in HP
• Apply to individual spot and hold in place for at least 5 minutes

I did this on the couch while watching a movie because it was a little time consuming. When my husband came home and saw the difference after two applications he yelled out loud (with joy for me :). The speed at which HP healed the remaining spots was astonishing. I literally could see it happening in the mirror. Toward the end of each of the three sessions, spots I had started with were visibly reduced. So was the hyper pigmentation [...] and I went out WITHOUT FEELING HUMILIATED for the first time!"

Diabetes

Another area where Earth Clinic readers have expressed particularly encouraging results is with diabetes and pre-diabetic conditions. A number of ACV's virtuous components improve blood sugar control and provide relief from diabetes symptoms and secondary conditions. Foremost, we can be thankful that some of the enzymes in ACV help to process carbohydrates, moving sugar more effectively through the body and taking some of the responsibility off the shoulders of our natural insulin supplies.

The pectin in apples and ACV also helps to modulate blood sugar levels, preventing the dangerous sugar spikes that create long-term problems for diabetics. Among these secondary conditions are a number that result from circulation issues that can result in amputations and cardiovascular disease if left unchecked, but ACV helps to keep the vascular system loose and supple, encouraging blood flow to help prevent diabetic amputations and to keep the heart relaxed and strong.

Diarrhea

Apple cider vinegar kills off the pathogens that force the body to use diarrhea as a means to flush invading pathogens out, but it also brings the body back into balance when it is overreacting in those runaway cases of diarrhea that don't have a practical physiological cause. In regards to one of the primary causes of diarrhea, our readers consider it the number one, almost instant cure for food poisoning (see below).

> **Louise from Ocala, Florida:** "I had diarrhea (including blood) almost constantly for 8 1/2 weeks after a "holiday" party at work. I received the advice of 6 MD's, 1 nurse practitioner, & several public health nurses. I had lab tests done. Besides all that, I am a registered nurse. No one knew what was wrong with me (and yet they wanted to do even more expensive and invasive tests). I could eat only certain things. When I would take prescription medication - I had to keep taking it. Over the counter medication stopped the diarrhea but left me in constant pain and drowsiness. This week I was blessed to remember something I heard a long time ago about apple cider vinegar. So I tried a few mouthfuls. I had already had about 6 bowel movements that day. I didn't have any more problems that day (to my surprise) even though I had eaten alot. My only problem now is to fig-

ure out what should I eat first.. .a pizza, chocolate malt, grilled cheese with tomato? "

Chris from Romeo, Michigan: "My mom, 82, has bouts of diarrhea every month or so. This lasts for hours and hours and then slowly it subsides and next day she is okay. I remembered reading about taking ACV for this. I asked her if she would try it and she said yes. I mixed 2 tbsp of ACV (with the mother), and 1/4 tsp of baking soda (without aluminum, from the health food store) and about 8oz of water, and she drank it. She said immediately that she felt better. I checked on her about 15 minutes later and she said she was 100% better! I'm just elated! And so is she of course."

Eczema

Return your skin's pH balance to its natural state with a regular ACV wash — much less expensive than cosmetic products — and clear up those ugly, scratchy patches of eczema with remarkable speed. Add the ACV tonic (its potassium may address a deficiency that could be the root cause of eczema) and apple cider vinegar will work when no other remedy can.

Sean from Galway, Ireland: "Just started using ACV for eczema which had afflicted me for years now and the results are staggering. Had been previously using steroid creams for the condition but they only offered short-term respite. Anyway, while the ACV caused quite a stinging effect initially, it has allowed me some interrupted sleep for the first time in years."

Nvr2fit from Sacramento, California: "Apple Cider Vinegar has nearly cured my arms of eczema after only 3 days. I still have slightly bumpy forearms on the tops of both arms, but I am so amazed it is nearly gone. I took 1 tablespoon of ACV 3 times a day so far for 3 days and will continue for 7 more days for a total of 10 days. Incredible since 3 days ago the tops of my arms were enflamed incredibly itchy, unsightly red bumpy patches from my wrist to past my elbows. I have never given my testimonial about anything and had to for this because I am truly surprised it works so well and so fast! I was on the verge of picking up my prescription for Elidel which I knew would only mask the problem rather be the cure, but I was getting desperate as the eczema was spreading up my arm. On top of that with my insurance is costs $160! Bottom line, I'm a believer in the power and potency of ACV and encourage anyone to use it for their eczema."

Penelope from Toronto, Canada: "I have finally cured my eczema with ACV. I was reluctant to use it around my eyes and had been told to use cortisone creams sparingly as the eyelids are so sensitive. I was reluctant to try ACV but when I did - presto! Everything calmed down and now a week later, it seems that my problems with eczema are a thing of the past. I used about 1 Teaspoon diluted in a 1/2 cup of water. I applied it twice a day. Wonderful! Fabulous! Thanks so much."

Soh from Adelaide, Australia: "I was at my wit's end with eczema and inflamed skin. I had deep cuts and bleeding cracks on my right hand. I followed Earth Clinic's advice and applied ACV topically (store bought ACV) - it burnt but it stopped itching. I also started taking ACV internally twice a day (I do not mind the taste at all, I enjoy a glass of water with a tsp or two of ACV. Also, my headaches are gone and I feel refreshed and clear-headed and full of energy the whole day - we are talking peppy and clear headed after an 8 hour meeting here - the ACV is working wonders for me:) I have not had an itching episode for over a week now... and slowly but surely the hand is healing. "

Food Poisoning

We suggest that you drink two tablespoons straight apple cider vinegar the moment you feel you might have food poisoning. Of course, be prepared for your throat and stomach to burn a bit, but the relief after that is well worth the brief discomfort (and a cheap trade-off compared to days of nausea from food poisoning). You may even want to take the ACV tonic before going to a barbeque or any event where food may have been sitting around.

Mbs560 from Redwood City, California: "I had just returned from a long journey to Thailand and of all the exotic foods I ate along the way it was the last meal on the flight home that did me in. Feeling extremely nauseous with pangs of cramping I thought I could make my way through the next day using the old standby acidophilus yogurt cure. Not feeling any better after spending half the day vacillating between nausea, hunger and pain I searched the internet for a home remedy. Having heard Apple Cider Vinegar was an age-old use for just about everything including stain removal, I hopped in my car (still in my pj's) and took a Dixie cup full of vinegar, mixed it with half a cup of berry juice and downed the vile tasting swill. Even though I felt like vomiting right there in the store, I agree with a previous reader who said he could literally feeling it working. It felt as though all the bad bacteria were being "sizzled" in acid. It took about 45 minutes or so, but the cramping went away and I started to feel less nauseous. Unbelievable!!"

Deirdre from Los Angeles writes: "I took a shot's worth of straight apple cider vinegar the moment I got home from a restaurant and felt a queasy stomach from the chicken I had eaten. I usually dilute apple cider vinegar in water, but knew this time it had to go down straight if it was to work fast. Remarkably, it stopped my queasy stomach within 5 minutes. I am certain I did not get food poisoning because the apple cider vinegar quickly destroyed the bacteria in my colon and stomach. Amazing!"

Fungus

Nail fungus, athlete's foot, and other fungal infections can be embarrassing as well as uncomfortable, but fungi are very sensitive to the acid in ACV and can be defeated by an immune system strengthened with daily ACV tonics. Furthermore, many such infections can be traced back to specific nutrient deficiencies, and ACV can help the body to absorb more of those critical nutrients to repair the body's nutritional holes.

Thankful from Gurnee, Illinois: "I am in awe of the power of something as simple as apple cider vinegar. Two years ago I dropped a hairdryer on my right big toe. Apparently this was enough to cause an interruption in the nail bed where fungi developed. It started deceptively slowly with just a thin white strip on the side of the nail that was barely noticeable. My podiatrist didn't seem particularly concerned about it, so neither was I. Besides, I typically wear nail polish and didn't have to look at it. However, at the beginning of this week I took my nail polish off and all the sudden I was the creature from the black lagoon! Eww!! Approximately 80% of my nail was funkified with yellow and white globules, bumpy, thick and just gross. [...] I soaked my infected toe in full strength apple cider vinegar for 3 days equaling 30 minutes in the morning and 30 minutes at night. I saturated a piece of toilet paper with the ACV and just laid it on the nail while I watched TV. In just six treatments the infected part of my toenail fell off this afternoon with no pain whatsoever. Under the nail was the grossest wet sawdust-like substance I have ever seen. I can hardly believe the ACV worked so quickly to eradicate the ick. If someone would have told me that it would work this quickly I never would have believed it after everything I have read."

John from Dallas, Georgia: "I started the straight organic ACV soak for my athlete's foot (moccasin type) and toenail fungus after trying everything that is sold over the counter as well as one of the liver type pills to get rid of the fungus. Nothing worked. I had this foot fungus for at least 10 years, and I thought I was doomed to have this for the rest of my life until I found the EC website and decided to try soaking my feet in the organic ACV. I used it twice a day for three weeks and my athlete's foot has disappeared and I can see the new clear/white toenail growing in behind the thick/yellow one. Incredible stuff!"

Gas

Everyone deals with periods of gas that are both uncomfortable and embarrassing. ACV can restore the balance your body needs, promote healthy digestion, and reduce the process of fermentation that creates most of that gas and flatulence.

Marshall from Berkeley, California: "I've been having some horrible digestive trouble for weeks, and most recently began experiencing horrible gas pains every 15 minutes. The gas was trapped and would not come out either end. After 3 days of suffering, I decided to give ACV a try at this website's recommendation. GAS PAIN GONE! Almost instantly, the gas pains disappeared and I began farting and burping. I have never felt so grateful for flatulence!"

GERD

See **Acid Reflux** (above) for relief from this family of digestive disorders. Apple cider vinegar is far and away the most popular natural remedy we have found for GERD and other acid issues.

Gout

Here is another case where it seems to make a particular difference that you use organic, unfiltered and unpasteurized ACV to treat cases of gout, rather than a generic or processed vinegar. Here, the acid content of the vinegar is not enough. It is the complete spectrum of nutrients, probiotics, and prebiotics that contribute to a cure by promoting circulation of water and minerals throughout the body and dissolving the crystallized uric acid that creates the painful condition.

Barry from Shawnigan Lake, Canada: "I recently had my first bout with Gout, and ACV scored an impressive knockout! I had been taking a diuretic for high blood pressure and in my initial research I learned that my medication could be contributing to my gout. It was New Years Eve and I couldn't get out to see my doctor until the following Monday (4 days later) [....] I followed the instructions on your website and began to take 2 tbsp with water, tomato juice, etc. Within 12 hours the swelling crested and within 36 hours I was about 80% better. I was completely cured within 5 days. My doctor confirmed that my medication could contribute to gout and was very impressed with ACV as a remedy. I decided to read up a little more about the benefits of ACV for my high blood pressure. Well, it's been 9 days now and with my doctors blessing, I've weaned myself off my medication. I've purchased an organic brand with the "mother" (available at most specialty grocery and health food stores) and I'm happy to report that my blood pressure is steady in the 122/80 range and is lower now that when I was on the medication (135/88). Thanks again! Like the old-timers, I've started to take it straight up (with an apple juice chaser) I have more energy and am continuing my daily routine of 1/2 shot glass 2-3 times a day as I attempt to shed 40 lbs over the next 6 months. It's the miracle I've been looking for and I'm telling the world!"

Robm from Las Vegas, Nevada: "I came down with a bad case of gout in my right big toe. I searched online and came across this site. I started by mixing 4 ounces of regular store bought apple cider vinegar with 20 ounces of cold water. I added a packet of sweetener to make it palatable. The next morning my pain had gone from an 8 to a 3 or 4. I continued with mixing 4 tablespoons of ACV with 8 ounces of water, 3x a day. It has now been 2 days and I am virtually pain free with full movement of my toe."

Bob from Dallas, Texas: "I had a Gout attack a few years back and remembered hearing about home remedies. Found a formula for 1 oz Apple Cider Vinegar (1 shot glass) in 1 cup hot water with a tsp of honey. Picked up the ACV at my local grocery store, fixed my ACV tea each evening while I watched TV, and the gout was gone in about 3 days. About a year later I was on a business trip and started developing symptoms so off to the store for ACV and this time nothing happened. I was upset and could hardly walk through the airport. When I got home I looked at the ACV I had used before found it was organic. The stuff I picked up on my trip was from a local drug store and was distilled. Tried the formula with my organic and again the pain and swelling was gone in a couple of days."

Headache and Migraine

At its foundation, a headache is a sign of biological imbalance. The direct cause of pain is that the blood vessels in the brain are either constricted or dilated. The ACV tonic can help people who suffer from frequent headaches, such as migraines, by improving nutritional balance and working in its normal manner to relax and modulate vascular flow.

For acute headache pain – an actual headache or migraine attack – try inhaling a steamed 50/50 mixture of ACV and water. You don't need too much liquid, just pour the ACV and water into a pan and heat lightly over the stove. Place a towel over your head and bring your face over the mixture. Don't get the water too hot, and start slowly because the first breath of the ACV mixture can be strong.

More simply, lie back in a dark room and cover your forehead with a cloth soaked in ACV and water until the pain subsides.

Heart Conditions

The best treatment for heart conditions, particularly sudden chest pain, is to visit a doctor or emergency room. Nevertheless, ACV can offer some help in reducing and even reversing the long-term damage that we do to our hearts and cardiovascular system. In particular, ACV acts to reduce cholesterol levels, mitigate hypertension, and improve the nutritional resources available for the body's own self-maintenance tasks. Furthermore, its antioxidants help prevent further damage to heart tissue, and as a muscle the heart is particularly sensitive to the body's lack of potassium, which ACV can help to restore.

Heartburn

Please see reader feedback at **Acid Reflux**.

High Cholesterol

The water soluble pectin in ACV is an excellent form of fiber that binds with cholesterol and sweeps it out of your system, while the antioxidant components of ACV prevent the oxidation of cholesterol into charged cholesterol molecules that are even more dangerous.

Sathiananthen from Singapore: "I have been taking ACV for some time now. Reason, high cholesterol and so on. My reading taken on 23/10/09: Cholesterol 7.73, Triglycerides 1.33, HDL-C 0.94, LDL-C 6.19 and Chol: HDL Ratio 8.22 all in mmol/L measurement. I went on an offensive with ACV 2 cap full, lemon juice 2 teaspoons and 1 teaspoon of honey with piping hot water, drinking slowly.

Current result taken on 07/01/2010: Cholesterol 4.63, Triglycerides 1.55, HDL-C 1.05, LDL-C 2.88 and Chol: HDL Ratio 4.41 all in mmol/L. For me it works well but in terms of losing weight I don't see much. I introduced ACV to my manager who has the same problem and never once has seen his results pass the cholesterol test. After my advice and 3 or 4 weeks of taking ACV on a daily basis, last week's results outshine even my report."

Hives

The sudden onset of hives signals the body's intense effort to get rid of a pathogen and bring the body back into balance. An ACV wash can kill many of these pathogens and restore the skin's natural state while relieving the itch and irritation.

Jamie from San Jose, California: "Recently I used indoor tanning cream (for a tanning bed) [which gave me a] tingle on my legs and arms. I got home and showered and was so itchy and blotchy I called in sick to work. I applied ACV with a cotton pad twice directly to my legs and arms and within about 8 minutes the pain and redness was completely gone!!"

IBS (Irritable Bowel Syndrome)

IBS is another condition with an increasing incidence rate that modern medicine has not been able to explain or address to anyone's satisfaction, but as with other digestive disorders a number of our readers have reported relief by using ACV when they couldn't find reliable help anywhere else.

> **Lillian from Chicago, Illinois:** "Have been having severe IBS-D symptoms for the past week and on and off for months--nothing has helped, except sometimes peppermint. Finally decided to give apple cider vinegar a try, since it's so highly thought of. Stirred a tablespoon into a glass of water with a little cinnamon and ground ginger, plus the tiniest drop of honey. Not only was it delicious, but my stomach feels great for the first time today."

Joint Pain

As with gout, joint pain in general is often caused by accumulations of minerals that form accretions on bones, joints, and connective tissue. It's these accumulated minerals that cause joint pain and stiffness, and bringing ACV into your regular diet has been proven to dissolve and reduce such deposits not only in our veins and arteries but throughout the body as well by restoring needed pH values and by increasing intercellular and intracellular circulation of water, waste, and nutrients.

> **Natural Girl from North Carolina:** "I stumbled across EC in my desperation to relieve a really bad flare up of joint pain & inflammation a couple of months ago and I haven't had my nose out of this site much since! I started with adding a splash of ACV to my drinking water (I try to get my 8 glasses a day). Thought it can't hurt to try it. Was really surprised at how much relief it provided. Don't

think I'll ever be without it now. Wish I had some idea what causes these flare-ups. [...] For now though, I think every 'body' needs a little ACV daily! "

Suzanne from Abbotsford, British Columbia: "I took glucosamine sulphate for my joints for many years because it helped. Then when I had frozen shoulder, I took a supplement in the hopes that it would help. It made me feel young again, except for my shoulder. However, I found it to be too expensive for me, so when I read about ACV on this website, I decided to try it. I only take 1 tablespoon a day with a glass of water, but that is enough for my joints to feel ok. Sometimes I add 1/4 t. baking soda, esp. if I feel like I'm "coming down" with something. Then I might make a tonic of a couple of tablespoons ACV, lemon juice, and honey, mixed in a mug of hot water. Every week I skip a day or two, as that was recommended somewhere on here."

Menstrual Issues

Throw a cup of ACV in your bathwater to ease cramping during your menstrual period, and use the ACV tonic to keep your system nourished and in balance.

Somewhereinchina from Beijing, China: "When I hadn't had my period for 6 months (not preggers), I thought I may have to go to a doc. Then I saw this site! I drank Apple cider vinegar for 2 days - one 8 oz. glass of water with 3 tablespoons once in AM, once in PM. My period just came! I'm a believer!"

Christy from Mechanicsburg, Pennsylvania: "I want to add my voice to the chorus of "YAY ACV!!" I had horrible cramps - once so bad I went to the ER worrying something was very wrong. They did an examination AND an ultrasound and found nothing. I bled so much that I couldn't go to work because I'd be useless there. It was really horrible.

I saw all these sites about supplements and things and I am not one for the holistic approach. I took my Advil or muscle relaxers anything really just to stop the pain - but of course they made me bleed worse. So when I tried ACV I was astounded! I have often said - short of a miraculous healing, I have never ever seen something work so well! My bleeding all but stopped. My cramps went AWAY!!! I can't even begin to tell you of the relief! [...] I've been using ACV for about 7 months now and every time I use it - it works like a charm. I need to make sure to start drinking it before my period, or I do have a day of groaning while I wait for it to take effect.

I usually took 1 tablespoon with an 8oz glass of water, juice, tea etc - but lately I've been adding it to a full sized bottle of tea or juice and kinda eyeballing it. Still works though I'm thinking I should probably start measuring again just to control the amount of acid going into my stomach."

Moles

Scratch at the outer surface of any mole on your skin, dab it with ACV, apply a band-aid, repeat, and within surprisingly few days the mole that has forever been a blemish upon your appearance may be entirely gone. Of course, talk to a doctor about any mole that appears, grows, or changes shape suddenly to rule out the possibility of skin cancer.

Bonnie from Manlius, New York: "Ok, so I decided to rid myself of a very unattractive mole on the left side of my face, on my hairline. I brought my trusty bottle of ACV to work (yes, work... I'm not so inclined to slap a piece of duct tape on my face to secure a stinky piece of acv soaked cotton while trying to sleep). Sitting cautiously behind my computer, so as not to pique the curiosity of my co-workers, I soaked a q-tip in the acv and applied it directly to the mole. I then sat and read Earth Clinic posts for ten minutes or so (hope the IT staff were on break). I started this self-inflicted facial hooplah three days ago and only did it once a day and today... it's gone! Of course, it looked like I had a science experiment growing on the side of my face for a couple days! It enlarged and turned blood red on day one, as if it were going to put up a fight (puh-LEEZE) and then it scabbed up and turned black the following day. As I read it it's last rites, it simply fell off! I swear I heard it whisper "I'll beee baaack" but ain't NO MOLE strong enough to withstand the power of pure, undiluted acv!"

Dredot from Asheville, North Carolina: "First of all, I was skeptical Apple Cider Vinegar would work- I'm not going to lie! But over the last six years I had seen two dermatologists about a mole on the very end of my nose. Both of them tried to remove the mole by means of freezing, and shaving. Both times it came back. It's been quite the journey for that little guy... but I really wanted to get rid of him. So, I gave ACV a try after reading this site. Started the regime a little over a week ago with scratching the mole with the broken end of a toothpick, essentially roughing up the surface a little, then applied a cotton swap about the same size of the mole soaked in ACV over it and applied a band-aid to hold it in place over night. Did this three nights in a row. The first day it bubbled a little. Nothing too noticeable. Second day after I took off the band-aid in the am, it has scabbed over looking black (just like everyone said it would). The third day I took a hot shower and afterward I peeled the scab right off and it left a crater-sized hole. Honestly, I looked like a mess - but I prevailed and by the fourth day I could already see the damaged skin reviving itself and starting to heal. Today its day 8 and you can hardly see anything. My skin is looking healthy. I'm thrilled!"

Brian from Staten Island, New York: "I recently read about Castor Cream and Apple Cider Vinegar used for removing moles, so I tried one of each on two different moles on my neck. I applied both for a couple of hours each day for about two weeks (using a soaked cotton pad of ACV, held with a Band-Aid, and simply applying the

Castor Oil with Baking Soda on the other). While the castor cream seems to have little effect, the ACV definitely worked. A couple of days after the tip of the mole scabbed I felt the mole with my hand, scratched it a bit and it felt as if the scab just fell off. I went to check it in the mirror to find that the whole mole itself actually fell off! ACV definitely works for mole removal."

PMS

As with other menstrual issues (see above), ACV can help your body maintain homeostasis when changes in hormone levels are upsetting your balance. Try blackstrap molasses as a sweetener for even more PMS relief.

Stephanie from Orlando, Florida: "I started to take ACV and baking soda about a month ago. My reasoning is for my PMS, it has been progressively been getting worse over the past year. I really didn't want to go back on birth control since it made me gain weight. I am happy to say that I have had no cramps, bloating, or chest swelling and it came a week early. Plus another bonus is that I have lost some weight. My emotional levels were so up and down I felt like I was going crazy during my period. And for the first time ever! I feel normal during my period. Thank you so much I would have not known about this cure without this site! My recipe is 2 tablespoons of ACV and 1 tsp of baking soda with 10 oz of cold water once a day."

Rosacea

The very public embarrassment of rosacea's reddening of the skin around your face can be relieved by dietary intake of ACV, which will improve circulation problems beneath the skin and bring the skin's chemistry back into balance on the surface.

Mike from Yakima, Washington: "I came across your site while looking for a cure. They say there is none. Have been mixing 1 tablespoon of ACV with a glass of water 2 times a day. Results have been incredible in the two plus weeks. Skin on nose has smoothed out--no breakouts. Redness is gone. Skin feels moist and smooth all over. Always tried topical treatments, which would cause dryness. Works for me, hope it helps others. Mental outlook as well as overall physical has improved."

Shingles

Painful shingles outbreaks can be miserable, and pain from the viral outbreak can last for months and years after the rash has disappeared. It's a condition modern science understands very little about and for which it can offer little relief, but our readers report excellent results from an ACV wash on the rash and pain relief from continued drinking of the ACV tonic. For an immediate way to ease the pain, use a cloth to apply ACV directly on the aching rash.

Jamie from Indianapolis, Indiana: "I tried the ACV after reading testimonials. It relieved the pain and the rash is clearing. I did go to the doctor and am on medication but the ACV really does help."

H from Bixby, Oklahoma: "Developed my first case of the shingles after minor surgery! Ouch! They're worse than surgery! And itchy!!! After going several days just using the Famciclovir the Dr. gave me and calamine lotion on the rash (about 3-4 nickel-quarter size 'bumps' which never formed blisters) I remembered Earth Clinic. The info provided here helped me with other conditions too!

Last night, this morning and this evening I drank 1 Tablespoon ACV in water with honey (heated up). Not exactly tasty, but I'll do what it takes. I also rubbed cotton balls soaked in ACV on the bumps several times. I'm still getting the shooting "pains" apparently associated with these shingles, but the bumps have already started to fade. It's already doing better than rubbing calamine 3-5 times a day!"

Sinus Issues

The tremendous pain of a sinus headache – whether from a sinus infection, allergies, or another ailment – is an imbalance that we feel like no other. Fungal and bacterial causes of sinusitis may be relieved by inhaling steamed ACV or with the use of a Neti pot nasal wash. The ACV tonic can address internal causes.

Cindy from San Diego, California: "I am 58 this year and for years have "suffered" from sinus issues. Now, it seems that I cannot have a good night's sleep because I usually wake up with terrible sinus pressure above my eyebrows. I have been on antibiotics twice since December. I hadn't read anything lately about ACV but remembered my grandfather always had a bottle in the bathroom and mixed it with baking soda and water. Because I was a child I didn't take note of the quantities. Last night, after searching the house for something to take for the horrible headache, I remembered the "concoction" (maybe grandpa from the grave?) Anyway, I poured a little into a glass and slugged it straight. No water and no baking soda. Immediately my eyes teared and my throat got phlegmy I coughed and my nose began to run... and run and run and soon, no headache! So this morning I got up and wanted to search for the "recipe." I read yours and now I hope that I will finally get a good night's rest."

Jnd2008 from Central New York: "I'm on my knees sneezing really thick deep green things that fill a towel and thinking of a doctors visit. Then I found this site. Read a bunch and came a crossed ACV mixes for flushing the sinus. A good friend told me about Apple Cider

Vinegar once, and how it helps the body. Picked up a Neti Pot (under $20), which came with a bunch of pre-mixed packets. I just grabbed the Neti Pot and mixed 8oz of warm water with 1 tablespoon of ACV with a big pitch of salt. Poured through nose with no pain until 1/2 hour later. One molar right side went crazy (pain) all the way to the root tip. As well as sneezing while it drained. Two Advil to reduce pain. Fell asleep for 3 hours.

Made a second batch, 8oz warm water 1 tablespoon of ACV plus another 1/2 tablespoon of ACV for good measure, no salt. Complete flush with no pain during or later. 1 hour later sneezing is only clear fluid. Molar has totally subsided to normal and I feel great in a 20-hour span from the first flush to right now. I'm totally impressed and will be passing this on to all."

Wendie from Phoenix, Arizona: "I've had a sinus infection for 2 weeks - super painful. I didn't know what to do. I saw on your site about ACV and did your suggested measurements of 2 tablespoons ACV with 8 oz warm water 3x a day for 24hrs. Almost to the hour I was breathing really clearly and my sense of smell was coming back! I am so excited about this."

Reinventyourhealth from Redding, California: "I am a 53 yr old male and I have had sinus problems periodically for 10 years. Lately, they have been getting progressively worse and much more severe. The deciding factor for me to try one of the suggested remedies was when, just a few days ago, I experienced severe sinus blockage on the left side of my face and what I initially thought to be some dental problems as my cheek was swollen from the impacted sinus cavity. Anyway, I scanned the various remedies and tried the 50/50 mixture of ACV and purified water. I mixed up the solution and put it into an unused nasal mister bottle. The suggestion was to pump 4-5 sprays in to each nostril. I knew it would sting with the 5% acidity of the ACV so I opted for 1 pump in each nostril to start. I was glad I did as it definitely stings for approx. 10 sec. I also chose to sniff my nose to get it further in to the blocked sinuses. If you can tough out the stinging, you should be quite pleased with the results. I actually ended up doing

4 pumps in each nostril just not all at once. Within a half hour my sinuses were starting to open up and the pain was subsiding in the upper jaw. Approximately 3 hours later and I was able to breath through my left nostril that was previously blocked. I can testify to the effectiveness of this treatment as it really cleared me up and saved me tremendous medical costs as this solution cost less than 25 cents to mix."

Arlene from Meredosia, Illinois: "I just realized after two weeks of ACV, not only all of my sinus problems are gone, but the muscle aches that accompanied it. I didn't realize that that was what was causing the pain all over my body until someone mentioned it on this site. My husband and I have been miserable with the sinus headaches, congestion etc., but we attributed the aches and pains to arthritis. We are in our 70's so it was logical. It wasn't arthritis at all it was the sinus infection. I feel 100% better."

Skin Issues

ACV can improve your skin inside and out, restoring your skin's natural acidity that soaps can strip away, clearing up skin conditions, and restoring a youthful glow and skin tone all over. It's a veritable Fountain of Youth!

Harbo from San Diego, California: "I take two teaspoons of apple cider vinegar to 8oz of water every other day and I have noticed a STRONG difference in my body. I developed "nummular eczema" on my legs over three years ago, which prevents me from shaving from the knees down. My legs were constantly breaking out and the bumps would flare if I went to a dry city, keeping me awake all night in itchy pain. Lotion, baby oils, topical medicated creams, you name it, I used it. But since I've been using raw ACV I no longer suffer from blotchy red bumps on my legs and am free to shave every day!! It's absolutely amazing and something that three different doctors couldn't cure or even treat. The mild detoxification that the ACV did was truly remarkable and I will continue using it for the rest of my life!"

Carrie from Denver, Colorado: "I have been using a facial toner of 1/2 ACV and 1/2 water, put into a small spray bottle. I spray this on my face in the mornings and evenings. Every other day, I exfoliate my face with baking soda. I have seen a big difference! My skin tone is even, pores are much smaller, and skin looks great! The only drawback is that others in my household don't appreciate the smell of vinegar wafting thru the air."

Sore Throat

For sore throats, our readers recommend a stronger concentration of ACV, up to 2 tablespoons with water and sometimes even more. The first few sips are likely to sting, but after that relief is quick to arrive and long lasting. Some readers add a dash of cayenne pepper and report outstanding results.

West from Dunn, North Carolina: "Whenever I start feeling a sore throat coming on I take a teaspoon of ACV and again in about 30 minutes. Soon after, my symptoms are gone. Also if you mix a teaspoon of ACV with a teaspoon of honey in a cup of tea, heat and drink, it will not only give you more energy but also help your sore throat feel much better."

Kyrt from Los Angeles, California: "ACV is awesome. I'm on day two of a sore throat. My voice sounded like a cartoon character. Found this site, hit the ACV, and no joke, it's only been 10 minutes, but my voice is back to normal. Guess what I'm drinking all nite :)"

Feeling Better Already from Northland, New Zealand: "I have to say that ACV diluted with warm water worked for me. The usual story, woke with an awful sore throat & couldn't swallow without feeling like I had sandpaper at the back of my throat. I remembered someone else mentioning ages ago that ACV helps. I hunted out a bottle that's probably been in the pantry since the beginning of time and I tried it. And you know what.? It works! First dose I knocked back 'straight' (ugh..!) Wow - needed a warm water chaser then. Am now sipping it with diluted warm water & will continue throughout the day. Sore throat has not completely gone as yet, but definitely feeling so much better. I can actually swallow without cringing. It almost seems to have an anaesthetic effect too. I smell like a pickled onion, but more importantly, I can breathe & swallow & actually function almost normally. Great stuff I say! No more pharmacies & docs for me when I get a sore throat!"

Mina from Little Rock, Arkansas: "I found myself looking for some feedback on this remedy, was having a lot of discomfort with the sore throat. I used the 3 tsp of apple cider vinegar, 3 tsp of honey, with about 8 oz of warm cinnamon tea, and then added just the tip of the tsp, less than 1/4 of cayenne pepper and gargle then drank the tea. It actually tasted good, I sipped it for about 10 min, now I can swallow my saliva and can go back to sleep!"

Warts

A lot of interesting tales are spun around sure-fire home remedies for warts, but ACV seems to really work. In this case, it is largely the acid that is killing off the virus that causes warts. That's the same case as with the common commercial treatment for warts, salicylic acid, except that the commercial treatment is more toxic to surrounding tissues.

Sonal from Charlotte, North Carolina: "I had a wart on my chin and recently applied vinegar on cotton ball at night and secured it with bandage. It's gone in 3 days. Can't believe it's actually gone."

Pacheco Family from Sedona, Arizona: "My son developed a wart on his foot that was starting to hurt him. As I work in an integrative health library I saw that ACV worked to kill the wart. I would prop him up in bed and soak the wart in ACV for 30 minutes. I would then attach a cottonball soaked in ACV to his foot with duct tape, put a sock over it and have him sleep with it on. Removing it in the morning and placing a band-aid on it for the day to keep clean. I did this every night for 3 days and saw a HUGE improvement. We were able to clean it out and even remove the dead skin. Within the week the wart was dead and not there is only a small mark where it used to be. AMAZING! "

Erin from Tuttle, Oklahoma: "I had a wart on my pinky finger for 4 years. I used the freeze off wart remover kits you can buy at the store and they got rid of it, but it kept coming back with a vengeance. My sister mentioned this website and I decided to try the ACV cure. I soaked a cotton ball in ACV and secured it to the wart with a bandaid before bed. I'm not going to lie, it hurt really bad... but I figured that's how I knew it was working. The only way I can describe the pain is, it was like someone was trying to drive a phillip's head screwdriver through my pinky finger. In the morning, I would remove the cotton ball and bandaid and repeat at night. The hard, rough bump came off in a few days, but that sucker was deep! I'm a "picker" so I dug the black part (seed) out and continued with the ACV for a week. It's been 6 months and it has stayed completely gone."

Yeast Infection

Yet again, yeast infections seem to be inexplicably on the rise, and ACV is there to treat them when modern medical treatments come up short or are too toxic. ACV will kill the candida fungus at the base of a yeast infection or case of thrush while restoring balance to mucosal membranes and the typically acidic environments in the parts of our bodies where yeast infections often occur.

Virginia from Stillwater, Oklahoma: "After many, many rounds of antibiotics I got a horrible yeast infection (Candida Albicans). The itching was so intense that I couldn't sit down. I was pacing around my house. Never in my life have I had such intense itching! In desperation I grabbed a washcloth and poured a small amount (maybe 2 tablespoons of ACV) on it then ran the tap water over it briefly to saturate the cloth and held it on my genital area. The itching stopped IMMEDIATELY! No burning for me, just relief."

Jenn from Queens, New York: "I'm 28 yrs old and I found this site about a week ago in search of relief for a yeast infection. Sorry if this is TMI, but if this helps another person then so be it! I had extreme itching accompanied by sore rawness after that would just not go away. This went on for about 3-4 days, progressively getting worse. I used OTC Monistat 'one day treatment' that is supposed to be cleaner, faster working, and all together convenient, hence the title. Well I had relief, but only for 'ONE DAY'! The next morning I woke up itching again, so I googled the heck out of finding a natural remedy and found this amazing site.

I chose to try the ACV that the site recommended and just picked it up at my local grocery store. I also picked up a bottle of acidophilus capsules. The first night I honestly didn't even measure the first amount of ACV I diluted in a glass of water, as I was just desperate for something to work. Then I took an acidophilus capsule following the drink. Maybe it was just mentally expecting a difference but within about 30 minutes I felt like the itching decreased. So I drank another glass of AVC (minus the acidophilus) before bed (this time I measured about 2 tbsp in 8-10oz water) and by morning I was still slightly itchy but had decreased about 85%! On a side note my menstrual cycle had been extremely off for a few months, as this had been a high stress year for me, but my last period was in mid-October. Well that day, mid-afternoon I began spotting. Did I kill 2 birds with one stone? lol... Now I don't know if the AVC induced my period or if I got it regardless, but I will say that when I was a few hours late of taking my ACV I began to feel 'itchy' again, as I was taking the same dose (2 tbsp ACV in 8-10 oz water) once nightly.

It has been almost a week of the regimen I've been using and have had my period full-blown for about 4-5 days now. […] This is truly an amazing, healing solution. INCREDIBLE. I never thought I would be writing that my yeast infection is fully healed! No itching, burning, or discomfort anymore. I never realized how good ACV is for you. THANK YOU EARTH CLINIC!!!"

Chapter 5

A FEW LAST SONGS FROM THE ORCHARD

No doubt it's hard to believe the many claims that we make in this book, alongside our readers, for the effectiveness of apple cider vinegar treatments. In fact, we hear the very same claims of disbelief from people who write to the website—just before they continue on and explain how shocked they were when the claims turned out to be true in their own experience.

The fact of the matter is that ACV isn't really a cure for most of these conditions. The secret and the power of apple cider vinegar isn't in what it does to your stomach, the skin, or your muscles but in the way that it restores the body as a whole. ACV helps the human organism to work in the way that it is supposed to, providing the required nutrients and restoring the body's homeostasis so that your immune system, your digestive and excretory systems, and your skin do their jobs properly, and so that the metabolic processes that power your body and help restore and repair all of your cells and systems can keep all of those systems working properly.

So it s that within the specific apple cider vinegar remedies we talked about in the previous chapter (not to mention the many, many more to be found on www.EarthClinic.com), you may have noticed that ACV seems most effective at addressing a few particular areas of our health. These areas are the sort of big picture aspects of health, like the digestive and circulatory systems and their disorders. This is because daily ACV tonics improve nutritional uptake of vitamins and minerals, speeding up and streamlining the body's metabolism while keeping the body more balanced and effective in all its processes. Likewise, ACV helps to regulate the body's circulatory system, moving nutrients into and toxins out of the body through good hydration within and between our cells.

In this chapter we would like to take a few last looks at some of those larger concepts in health where ACV can play a singular role. However, before we dig deeply into some of the most promising rewards of regular ACV enjoyment, we should recognize that there are moments when caution should be taken in ACV use, and there are people for whom ACV is not the best bet for health.

ACV Warnings and Side Effects

As happy as we are with the ACV tonic and ACV treatments in general, caution should be taken with any medical treatment, even one as mild and natural as bringing apple cider vinegar into your daily diet. The most common complaints with the ACV tonic are headaches and indigestion. The latter is almost always caused by having taken too much ACV in a single dose or at the start of treatment, hoping for a quick remedy. Additionally, women sometimes experience increased menstrual bleeding, although in some cases this has been a welcome symptom where it had been lacking.

In one particular area of note, ACV can have an effect on thyroid function and can interfere with the uptake and metabolism of thyroid medicines. People undergoing short or long-term thyroid treatment are in the one group that we would most caution in regards to using internal ACV treatments. Some of our readers report that a gap of several hours between the ACV tonic and thyroid medications will eliminate the drug interaction, but please speak with your doctor on the matter.

More generally, two tips in particular should minimize or eliminate ACV side effects: **Start Slowly** and **Go Organic**.

We hope that you are as excited about ACV as we are, but we still caution that you should begin an ACV routine slowly. Allow the body to adjust, and you will get the best benefits. Start by using the minimum amount of ACV in the ACV tonic (one teaspoon will do) and then build up through the course of a week or two until you find the concentration and amount of ACV that your body prefers.

The second and most critical advice we can give to help avoid side effects and make the most of ACV is to expend the effort and moderately more money to use organic, unpasteurized ACV. In most cases, and for almost all internal uses, organic ACV is far more effective, causes fewer side effects, and is altogether superior. Organic ACV simply provides food the way nature intended it and the way the body is prepared to accept it. If you have had minor side effects when drinking processed apple cider vinegar, organic ACV may treat you much better.

Pasteurization of apple cider vinegar requires temperatures between 140 and 160° F. That's hot enough to kill acetobacter bacteria, stop the acetification process, and prevent the growth of dangerous bacteria; but it also ends up killing others sorts of both good bacteria in the raw ACV mix.

How you take ACV can indeed make a difference in how well it relieves your condition and whether or not you experience side effects. One particular concern with ACV, where in truth we're inclined to say an emphatic "No", is with ACV capsules. People who dislike the initial taste of vinegar have written to us asking about whether the capsules of dehydrated apple cider vinegar available in some health stores would be a good shortcut to get past the taste of the ACV tonic. Our position at Earth Clinic is that there are very few shortcuts to health that are very good for us in the long run, and this easy-way-out strategy could be particularly ill advised. There are several disturbing reports of ACV capsule users who needed difficult treatment for severe throat burns when their ACV capsule became lodged and then dissolved in their throat. Moreover, ACV capsules offer a very concentrated dose of ACV, whereas everything we are finding points to the benefits of a mild and continuing ACV dosage in cases other than food poisoning. After all, we want to bring the body into balance, not shock it into submission.

Occasionally our readers have reported side effects that actually sound like and sometimes turn out to be rather good things. What we mean is that the healing process itself can create side effects. In particular, many of our readers have found that if you have a yeast infection your body may react with a wide range of secondary effects once you begin ACV treatment. This can be a good sign. The body often goes through a period when symptoms worsen as a part of what is called a "healing crisis" caused by the release of toxins created by the condition but stored away in the body (often in the body's fatty tissue). The effect here is much like how a fever will get continually worse until it at last breaks and the sick person thereafter begins to rapidly recover. This healing crisis is well documented and also called a Herxheimer Reaction. In this case, you may want to push through your side effects as a necessary step in healing, but each case of this sort should be examined individually.

In the end, if you feel that ACV treatment of any kind is causing side effects, look for another remedy and stop using the ACV. As we have said, ACV is not a cure-all and not the right remedy for every person or in every situation. Each person's health is complicated even at the best of times, and we cannot rely on any single remedy to cure all ills.

At the very least, it is best for everyone, even those who respond most positively to ACV treatments, to take a break from ACV occasionally. If you are taking ACV three times a day, consider a six-day-a-week treatment, going one day without to let the body readjust. This should help you avoid any side effects from long-term use.

ACV and Dental Enamel

Much has been made about dental concerns in regards to regular use of apple cider vinegar. Our readers sometimes worry that taking the ACV tonic as much as three times a day will begin to erode the enamel on their teeth and lead to cavities. This is definitely a legitimate concern, and people have chosen to drink their tonics through a straw in order to avoid the teeth. Others take a shot of ACV straight back and then wash the mouth out with water immediately afterwards.

We definitely recommend that you either drink water immediately after your ACV tonic (most likely you aren't getting enough water in your diet anyhow), or that you drink the highly diluted version of the tonic that we recommend for drinking throughout the day.

On the other hand, the risk shouldn't be exaggerated. The ACV tonic is in fact almost certainly less damaging to your teeth than the sodas many of us drink without a second thought. The pH value of undiluted ACV is about 2.4, very comparable to colas at a pH of 2.5. Other sodas tend to run in a pH range from 2.3-3.3 and are made worse by high concentrations of sugar that make the acidic soda's effects on dental enamel and dentin even worse, since natural bacteria in your mouth convert that sugar into additional acid. Meanwhile, if you are drinking one tablespoon of ACV diluted in 8oz of water (the highest recommended concentration), the acidity of your ACV tonic is diluted to a pH of about 3.0. That's substantially less acidic than your Coke or Pepsi and equal to a glass of orange juice. In other words, if you are drinking both ACV and carbonated beverages all day long, you should be concerned about your teeth. Otherwise, simply keep up a normal dental care routine.

ACV for Weight Loss

In getting back to the plus side of ACV, we know that in looking for its benefits most of us have to temper our desire for immediate results. The potential benefit of good general health and the promise of a long and active life are great motivations for picking up the apple cider vinegar habit, but they're also a bit too intangible to really grab onto. In truth, it's hard enough to plan our lives a week ahead let alone to give really serious thought about how we're going to be living when we're 80 and whether we're likely to make it to 85.

Yet many of us are plenty excited right here and now about the possibility that apple cider vinegar might help us to lose weight — and to keep it off — with a pleasant beverage rather than another miserable sit-up.

Even when they were looking for something entirely different out of their use of the ACV tonic, our readers have found themselves experiencing surprising and sometimes long-sought weight loss results with no other changes to their diet or exercise routines. For certain, without a proper diet and some level of exercise we cannot reach or maintain our ideal body weights, but ACV seems able to quickly launch us toward better metabolic functioning and a reduction in overall body fat, as Amy from Chicago, Illinois found:

> "Last summer, I was using apple cider vinegar on a daily basis to treat some persistent heartburn. I noticed that I lost about ten pounds over the course of six weeks. The change was so noticeable that my mother (who is usually quite critical of my weight) expressed concern that I had become too thin! By the winter, though, I had stopped taking the apple cider vinegar, and the weight had all come back. It never occurred to me that my weight loss had been due to the vinegar. Recently, I came across your website and decided to start drinking vinegar on a regular basis for overall health. It's been two weeks, and I'm already down four pounds! I've noticed that I seem to crave "bad" foods much less, and I am satisfied with smaller portions. Maybe that's due to the apple cider vinegar, or maybe it's just psychosomatic. Either way, I'm going to keep it up!"

A few theories make sense as to how ACV is helping us lose weight, and these ideas have been backed up by repeated research. First of all, ACV helps the body to draw out and use more of the available nutrition in the foods we eat. With our needs met, we feel fewer cravings to eat more than we should, and multiple studies have indeed found that vinegar increases the body's feeling of satiety.

Secondly, acetic acid helps in the metabolism of fats, breaking them down into their constituent parts and converting those fats into energy that helps keep us alert and active, giving us energy while keeping the weight from piling onto our middles. Japanese researchers doing acetic acid research on mice published a study in 2009 with the supposition that vinegar may be turning on fatty acid oxidizing enzymes and the genes that code them. Simultaneously, acetic acid can pass directly from our digestive track into our veins, where it also plays a role in releasing the energy from carbohydrates, helping the body burn calories efficiently.

Cholesterol is a sort of collection of fats, and despite its bad reputation it is essential to several biological processes. Unfortunately, it is very easy to accumulate more cholesterol in the body than is needed, and when we have too much waxy cholesterol it becomes a major part of atherosclerosis, as it can build up on cell walls and restrict blood flow.

Those findings may lend credence to the potential of the popular and seemingly effective Mediterranean Diet, which incorporates vinegar heavily into its menu, helping to make each bite of food more full of nutrients. Thus every calorie is used to its fullest so that in the end dieters can take fewer bites and consume fewer calories. Regardless of the exact mechanisms that ACV brings to bear on our weight loss efforts, it works and is improving our health in other areas while we lose the pounds. Of course, losing those pounds will in turn improve our health. As Crazydogjack from New Castle, Pennsylvania says, ACV is so good for you in general that weight loss is just a bonus:

> "I have lost a total of 16.5 lbs. to date! I do not crave sweets and I have a lot more energy. I am eating smaller portions as well. Those of you trying this for weight loss don't give up... stick with it. There are so many other positive benefits to ACV so drink it anyway!"

ACV and Fatigue

Efficient metabolism and proper, full use of the nutrition we bring into our bodies again plays a role in what ACV can offer those of us who find ourselves continually fatigued, fuzzy in the brain, and lacking energy to match our enthusiasm for life and to energetically pursue all the good things we could be doing if only we didn't feel so tired all the time. Lack of potassium is one frequent cause of lethargy and fatigue, and we've talked about the supply of potassium ACV provides. We've also just talked about how ACV can break down fats (our most potent energy source) and help to efficiently metabolize sugars in the bloodstream. The results our readers and formal medical studies have reported on the ability of vinegar to help diabetic conditions – modulating blood sugar levels and improving carbohydrate management in the body – are probably related issues, all part of how ACV can help the body's power plants keep a strong, even flow of energy through the body.

Of course, that flow is sometimes impeded by toxins, including those taken in from our poisoned environment, but we even produce toxins when we metabolize our foods. These toxins can interrupt metabolic processes and slow the body down, robbing us of energy on a continuing basis. ACV addresses this malfunctioning of our health by serving as a detoxifying agent, sweeping up free radicals that damage bodily cells, breaking down pathogens, and helping the body to expel poisons more easily via smooth and copious blood flow. When the body no longer needs to fight constant battles in breaking down and isolating these toxins within the body, it can devote more of your energy to the outside world and the things we love to do.

One repeated recommendation to combat fatigue is a simple recipe of baked beans and apple cider vinegar. Dr. Jarvis recommended it to his patients to add energy to their lives, and our readers on their own have made the same recommendation. This combination offers even more potassium for energy and muscle function while contributing a good supply of iron as well to combat anemia and help carry energy-creating oxygen in the blood.

Probiotics and their sister prebiotics are relatively new players as identified in the field of health, with as much promise as uncertainty. They are microorganisms, such as the live cultures to be found in yogurt, that do a host of things within and for our bodies. Some of the probiotics in ACV help in digestion, others may help combat pathogenic microorganisms, and some probiotics help in producing or making available vitamins and minerals that our bodies need.

ACV and Baking Soda

Not so very long after a burst of ACV energy got the Earth Clinic website rocking, our community made the happy acquaintance of a man we know as Ted, and with good reason. We know him as Ted for the simple reason that most of us have trouble with his given name, Parhatsathid Nabadalung, but it's with good reason that we have come to know him so well. Ted, a resident and son of Bangkok, Thailand has become our own resident consultant on many of the most popular remedies Earth Clinic has explored, particularly in the areas of the body's alkaline/acid balance. Ted came to his expertise in natural medicine beginning very early in his youth, inspired by his own and his family's medical needs and the remarkable relief and life-saving results they found in simple remedies such as Vitamin C and baking soda.

Through his generosity we have all come to benefit from Ted's lifelong passion for modern folk medicine, which has been expanded through wide-ranging medical education, and by his continuing medical experiments with his own health and the health of the many people who consult with him on their conditions and general wellness needs. We have come to trust and rely on him for expanding our community's overall medical knowledge and understanding, but in particular he has studied the benefits of baking soda or sodium bicarbonate for our health. Over the years with us he has refined and perfected a combined ACV and Baking Soda treatment that has been answered with great applause from our community, and which we will leave to Ted to explain here.

FROM TED

The apple cider vinegar and baking soda remedy was created to resolve a couple of problems concerning apple cider vinegar, primarily that it causes stomach upsets, which I have identified to be caused by the acidity of the ACV. The addition of baking soda to the ACV tonic also increases the antioxidant value, supporting the body's redox balance, and answers the body's physiological need for bicarbonate. Baking soda was formulated to fill that need. When you add baking soda the pH of the apple cider vinegar tonic is raised close to a pH of 7.3 (from about a pH of 3), which is about the pH of the blood; and it's this alkalinity that is most compatible with the body.

If the pH levels of our foods are too different from the body's pH it tends to cause stress, resulting in stomach upset as well as other problems. The body requires a store of bicarbonate, which is mostly found in the pancreas, as it helps buffer pH changes like a shock absorber so that pH can be maintained at 7.35 much more easily. The pancreas controls insulin and hence blood glucose, so without sufficient bicarbonates pancreas function is affected. Several people who try to alkalize have observed when alkalizing themselves with baking soda added to apple cider vinegar that their urinary pH is increased to an ideal pH of neutral, or 7. I have seen too many instances of kidney damage, and this can always be predicted in people with a history of renal damage whenever their urinary pH falls below 5.5. The acidity of that urine literally digests the kidney, just the same as stomach acid digests the food we eat.

The redox reaction or reduction-oxidation reaction is complicated but absolutely essential to life. Redox chemical reactions involve a change in which atoms become either more positively or negatively charged, and this reaction happens everywhere. We see redox in the processes that make rust and fire, and the redox cycle provides our bodies with their energy. However, that creation of energy creates free radicals than can damage the cells of the body, so we need antioxidants to balance the redox cycle. This is what happens when you mix baking soda with apple cider vinegar. Without baking soda to neutralize ACV, the remedy becomes a pro-oxidant rather than an antioxidant. This phenomenon can easily be demonstrated with an ORP meter (Oxidation Reduction Potential meter), which measures the value of antioxidants in negative millivolts. Pro-oxidants, or simply oxidants, are measured in positive millivolts.

When adding baking soda to the apple cider vinegar tonic you are effectively converting an oxidant apple cider vinegar with an ORP value roughly above +200 millivolts to between -100 to -200 millivolts. About 90% of the foods we eat are acid forming, and nearly all foods and drinks are generally oxidative in nature, so they put stress on the body. This is why an alkalinity source is needed in the body. Whenever the body needs to mount a defense, for instance when there is an infection coming, the body will raise its alkalinity. This is because most bacteria and viruses tend to be active in the acidity range of your blood. Hence the body needs its alkalinity stores. For all of these reasons, I recommend the addition of baking soda to the ACV tonic.

The general remedy that I use is as follows:

2 tablespoons apple cider vinegar
1/2 teaspoon baking soda
Add water to between 1/2 to 1 glass

The water is required to dilute the mixture so that it will be more biologically compatible with the body. Children will tend to love taking baking soda with apple cider vinegar, because they like the fizz after you mix the two ingredients. So you get the best of both worlds, this tonic tastes good and has the best healing properties.

The apple cider vinegar contains two major components, which are acetic acid (found in vinegar) and malic acid, which is the apple acid. The acetic acid is anti-inflammatory while malic acid helps increase energy during the morning hours for those who want to find a replacement for caffeine in the morning.

Ideally the remedy is taken either before meals or after meals, and usually at least twice a day. It may reduce constipation, but for those who do have constipation even after taking the apple cider vinegar with baking soda, you may add 1/8 teaspoon of sea salt. I have found that whenever baking soda and sea salt are mixed, it has a laxative effect, but this only works for sea salt, not common table salt.

> In Thailand I have other people who really hate the smell of apple cider vinegar. In this event, I have to knock down the formula with some apple juice. The remedy is as follows:
>
> *2 tablespoons of apple juice*
> *1/2 teaspoon of baking soda*
> *Add water between 1/2 to 1 glass of water*
>
> This is a knock down version for those who don't like apple cider vinegar. Then there are people who simply can't afford apple cider vinegar, can't find it, and don't have time to ferment it. The rough formula in that case is as follows:
>
> *1 1/2 tablespoon of apple juice*
> *1/2 teaspoon baking soda*
> *1/4 teaspoon vinegar*
> *Add water between 1/2 to 1 glass of water*
>
> Mind you the above is not a perfect formula, but it has most of the properties of the apple cider vinegar less the organic compounds and the minerals found in the apple cider vinegar.

Any of Ted's remedies can provide you with the benefits of ACV while minimizing the possibility of stomach distress, protecting your teeth, and possibly offering even more antioxidant benefit.

ACV and Hair Care

One last personal benefit we shouldn't fail to mention is in the area of hair care. You may have already seen that we suggest ACV as a remedy for dandruff conditions, as Renee has found in Kingman, Arizona:

> "I've been using ACV as a hair rinse for decades. We keep a bottle of it in the shower with a plastic cup. After washing my hair, I dump about 1/2 cup ACV in the cup, fill with water, and then rinse my hair with it. I do not rinse again with plain water. The vinegar smell goes away when your hair dries and no, it does not change the color of your hair. I got my husband to try it years ago and he hasn't needed to use dandruff shampoo since — yay!"

She confirms what a lot of us have found, that even people with oily or normal hair can enjoy the benefits of an ACV wash as well. Its nutrients can refurbish hair, but in particular the acid breaks down overabundant oils and counteracts the negative side effects of most shampoos, which tend to be alkaline when the hair would prefer a slightly acidic mantle.

ACV and Pets

Personal benefit, however, isn't the limit of the natural, inexpensive good we can derive from ACV. Our pets, so dear to our lives and even our livelihoods, can benefit in nearly as many ways; and so far as we have found, every pet and farm animal can be treated by and enjoy ACV as we do. Many of Dr. Jarvis' revelations about ACV came from his studies of cows and horses. In fact he found that animals sought out ACV whenever possible and grew faster, healthier, and stronger when it was added to their regular diet. We have found the same.

Where Earth Clinic has the most to say about ACV and pets is with dogs, cats, and horses. While dairy farmers still make a fair bit of use of ACV for mastitis, as Dr. Jarvis long ago recommended, it seems that horse breeders and owners have taken the lead as ACV proponents on the world's farms. In fact, one of the top thoroughbred trainers in New Zealand, Australia, and Oman wrote to say that he has been regularly feeding his top horses ACV, honey, and garlic for years with fantastic results and to the admiration of other trainers.

If you own horses, you may want to incorporate apple cider vinegar in your horse's diet in particular to combat the effects of arthritis. Additionally, a towel or bandage soaked in equal parts ACV and water can be wrapped around an arthritic joint or swollen limb and covered in plastic wrap for up to 3 or 4 hours to reduce swelling and pain. Most often, however, our readers throw a cup of ACV in the water barrel or 1/4 - 1/2 cup in a horse's daily grain feed for internal treatment with ACV. They find that the horse will eat better, drink more, have a better looking coat, can recover from injuries faster, and seems to improve in nearly every facet of health and activity. Most horses love the taste but are probably even happier to lose the biting flies. Horse owners find that ACV will help fend off flies and gnats, which don't like the taste of ACV in the horse's skin.

As with our human remedies, readers report that ACV can bring about a swift cure where thousands of dollars worth of conventional medicines fail entirely. Still, whenever you begin to treat a condition in your pet with ACV, start with a very low dose in food or water and then increase the dose to whatever your pet will tolerate or enjoy. In this case, too much of a good thing is not a good thing. As a rule of thumb, we suggest that you take your pet's size into consideration most importantly, and try one teaspoon a day for a pet under 50 pounds. From there, slowly work your way upward in dosage. For skin application, mix ACV in a 1:1 solution with water so that the acid does not burn the skin.

Also around the barnyard, dairy farmers have long used ACV to treat mastitis in cows and goats, using about one tablespoon of ACV per animal in the morning feed. Unlike with typical penicillin treatments for mastitis, milk produced during this treatment period does not have to be discarded, and the results are excellent and long lasting. Dr. Jarvis was likewise impressed with these same results.

However, if you are a more typical pet owner there is still plenty of good health ACV can bring to your smaller pets. Dog and cat owners alike are thrilled to find that fleas and ticks are no fonder of the taste of ACV on your pet's skin than are the flies that find it distasteful in horses. Many pet owners entirely stop other flea and tick treatments. Instead, they add a bit of ACV to their pet's diet and then on about a weekly basis spray the pet down lightly with a spray bottle containing water and ACV in about a 6:1 mix. Insects don't like the smell or taste and so will wait for a better host than your dog or cat.

Now, if a skunk takes a similar but more active dislike to your dog or cat, skip the tomato juice or other home remedy for skunking and throw a quarter of a cup of ACV into bathwater to wash your pet down. Just a few minutes of washing will restore your pet's scent to an odor no worse than that of a fresh salad, and the results are long-lasting, unlike other treatments where your dog smells like skunk again as soon as it gets wet.

If you own a dog, grab the ACV bottle most especially if your canine suffers from arthritis. It will loosen up his joints and relieve arthritis pain just as it does for people. Dogs with allergies, particularly skin and food allergies, respond well to the addition of ACV to their food or water, and it has stopped the itching and scratching that has driven some pet owners crazy, even when months worth of other remedies brought no relief to either dog or owner. In particular, if your dog has rashes or red and raw skin, a topical application of ACV and water in equal parts can provide immediate relief and a lasting cure. For certain, that was Marianne's experience in Fayetteville, Arkansas:

> "My old dog has been plagued with some sort of skin problem for years. The constant biting, scratching, and licking has nearly driven me out of my mind. I was doing everything the Vet said, plus gentle baths, brushing, and washing her bed linens in special soaps. Then on Sunday I tried Apple Cider Vinegar. I used about 1/2 cup to a large glass of water. I poured it on her hips, tail area, upper and lower back. I noticed that she calmed down almost immediately. I have done the same thing on Monday and today, Tuesday. The dog is calm, sleeping and "thanking" me. I know she is saying, 'Thanks, you finally got something to kill those mites on me.'"

If your pet of choice is the cat, you and your cat are also likely to find relief from fleas and ticks with regular ACV use. In cats, however, our readers most commonly report positive results regarding eating issues and urinary disorders, including the common issue of finding crystals in your cat's urine. ACV can restore the proper levels of acidity to feline urine while helping the cat to eliminate calcium deposits that build up in the body and block the urinary tract.

A lot of our readers are also frustrated with the insufficiency and cheap contents of most commercial dog and cat foods. ACV can help your pet draw more nutrients out of those foods and bring the pet's body back into balance, avoiding the digestive and urinary disorders continued use of the same pet foods can cause.

The last thing we have to say is simply to listen to your pet. Your dog or cat won't know what it needs to make itself better, but it will know what its body likes. Try an ACV remedy on your pet. Most pets will eagerly seek out food and water with a bit of added ACV, but if your pet exhibits an aversion to the change consider either lowering the dose, switching the bowl (food or water) you mix the ACV into, or looking for another remedy altogether. Animals are often better attuned to their bodily needs than we are to our own.

Finding ACV Around the World

All these marvelous uses of apple cider vinegar demand a dependable source for ACV, and at an inexpensive price if possible. While vinegar in several varieties is usually available for sale at any local grocery store, apple cider vinegar can be harder to find, let alone the genuine organic ACV that we strongly advocate for in most circumstances.

In the United States, health food and organic food chains like Trader Joe's and Whole Foods are dependable sources of ACV, usually in a small choice of brands.

And while apples are more or less popular the world over, ACV can be harder to find in other parts of the world. The general rule of thumb is still to look first in organic foods and health food stores wherever you find yourself. After that, a few sources around the world seem to be your best bets.

- *In **Australia,** horse stables will buy apple cider vinegar in bulk for use with the horses. Horse supply companies or a local horse owner might be able to give you a lead on ACV sources.*

- *Readers report that the Bulk Barn in **Canada** offers organic ACV.*

- *American Garden is the most common brand of ACV in **India**. Pay close attention to whether the product is natural, complete, and unpasteurized.*

If local stores do not stock organic ACV, you might try local apple orchards or fruit sellers, which might produce their own ACV in limited supplies.

Lastly, the internet is always a source for those hard to find items, and you can search for a store that sells ACV in your area or go directly to the websites of companies whose brand of ACV you trust. They might ship bottles to you directly or help you find a store or distributor in your area.

Regardless of brand and where you find your apple cider vinegar, you can make a good guess about the quality of the bottle you are holding based on the color (it should be fairly dark) and the clarity (cloudy vinegar and solids at the bottom of the bottle indicate presence of the Mother). Then take a close look at the label to make sure the ACV you are holding is made from apples and not merely apple flavoring, has not been pasteurized or filtered, and is not a distilled product.

Make Your Own ACV

Of course, if you cannot find organic ACV in your part of town or the world, you can always make your own. The process is surprisingly low intensity and high in satisfaction. Complete guides are available to fully refine and expand your homemade ACV production, but we can give you a more than sufficient outline right here on the process of making apple cider vinegar, even in a crockpot on your kitchen counter.

There are only three steps to the production of apple cider vinegar, as with any vinegar. First, apples are used to make apple cider. Then apple cider is fermented to make hard apple cider. Lastly, the alcohol in hard apple cider is converted into acetic acid, making your apple cider vinegar. For the most part, this entire process will take place without our hardly lifting a finger.

For certain, making apple cider takes a bit of work. We're going to take it for granted that most of you are simply going to go to the store and purchase a gallon of apple cider or better yet get it straight from a local apple farm. The farm is in many cases the only chance you'll have of getting unpasteurized cider, which offers better nutritive value, but any apple cider will do (apple juice will not). If you choose to make your own cider, be certain to extract juice from every last bit of the apple—skin to seeds.

Now in getting from cider to hard cider to vinegar, the two things we need to be responsible for are temperature and oxygen. Most of the rest of the work we'll leave to nature.

1. *First, you want to transfer your cider to a glass, wooden, stainless steel, or enamel container for fermentation into the alcoholic hard apple cider. Other metals and plastics will leach metal and toxic compounds into your vinegar.*

   Your container should be no more than three-quarters full and it will need to be exposed to the air. It will be best if you leave any cover off the container and slip cheesecloth over the top to keep insects and dust out.

2. *Keep this container in a place away from direct sunlight and at room temperature (between 60-80 degrees F). Stir it once a day to keep the oxygen circulating.*

3. Yeast will naturally turn all of the cider's sugar into alcohol within about two weeks. Enough yeast exists naturally in the atmosphere to do the job, but if you would like to speed it along you can find brewing yeasts from a wine or beer making shop. Bread yeast is not a good substitute, better in that case to leave it to nature.

4. Once the sugars are converted to alcohol, nature will again take over and begin converting the alcohol molecules into acetic acid in the very same container. Again, you can accelerate this process by getting a bit of Mother of Vinegar from an old batch of ACV and adding it to your container once the fermentation process is complete, but that is unnecessary. Nature provides the acetobacter bacteria to do the job of acetification. Once the island of Mother of Vinegar has formed at the top of your maturing ACV, be gentle with the container and be careful not to knock the island around. You do not want it to fall down into the liquid, simply because the Mother will not do its work beneath the surface.

5. It will take about two more weeks after the fermentation process is complete, so about four weeks total, before the acetification is done and you have your finished homemade apple cider vinegar. Test your maturing vinegar daily to taste whether it has reached maturation.

6. At this point, you will want to scoop off the floating island of Mother of Vinegar at the top of your container and then filter the vinegar into your storage containers.

Cheesecloth or coffee filters will do the job nicely, cutting down the amount of cellulose fiber in the vinegar—those long strings of complex carbohydrates you are liable to see floating in your vinegar as it matures.

For the greatest safety, you could heat this newly made vinegar on the stove to between 140 and 160 degrees F to pasteurize the vinegar. However, we continue to recommend the unpasteurized vinegar, which has greater nutritive value. As an acid, vinegar is naturally antiseptic so there is little worry about your vinegar going bad, so long as you store it properly. Simply cap your containers and keep the vinegar out of direct sunlight. Room temperature storage is perfectly fine.

Additional Resources on the Website

To be frank, this book could only ever present the tip of the iceberg on apple cider vinegar. Our Earth Clinic website (www.EarthClinic.com) offers the full collection of our decade and more of ongoing conversations regarding ACV's many gifts. That ACV discussion is in the company of dozens of other natural remedies and forums for discussing a remarkable variety of physical and mental conditions that can be addressed by natural and folk medicine treatments. We invite you to become a part of that conversation and the Earth Clinic community.

As far as ACV is specifically concerned, you can find a lot more of the same on our website. Many people return to the site regularly for continually updated feedback in much greater number, more detail, and with a host of variations on how you can use ACV for any given condition. Likewise, you gain the company of so many others who have and currently are addressing the health concerns that worry you. The ailments we've listed in Chapter 4 are only the most common medical conditions and those best addressed by ACV, but the website has pages for dozens more conditions our readers have successfully addressed with the ACV tonic or ACV topical treatments.

Reader contributors have offered a whole collection of recipes to incorporate ACV into your diet, stories of inspiration to keep you on track in rejuvenating your life and conquering long-endured conditions, and constant updates on new ideas and successes in using ACV to make your health and your life the best they can be.

> *"I believe the doctor of the future will be a teacher as well as a physician. His real job will be to teach people how to be healthy. Doctors will be even busier than they are now because it is a lot harder to keep people well than it is just to get them over a sickness." Doctor D.C. Jarvis*

The best you can be and the healthiest version of yourself are our exact aims at Earth Clinic. Folk medicine for centuries has helped to promote and restore health, and modern medicine has more recently done wonders to fight back disease. We think the concept of modern folk medicine can bring a marriage of these two approaches to health and wellness, not just restoring health where it has gone wrong but going further and beginning to deny the claim that disease and sickness are inevitable. Modern folk medicine wants to assert that something like perfect health and wellness should be what we expect in life. Your own perfect picture of health is what modern folk medicine begins to offer and what apple cider vinegar strives to promote. We wish you the best in bringing that image to life.

Index

ABOUT THE AUTHORS

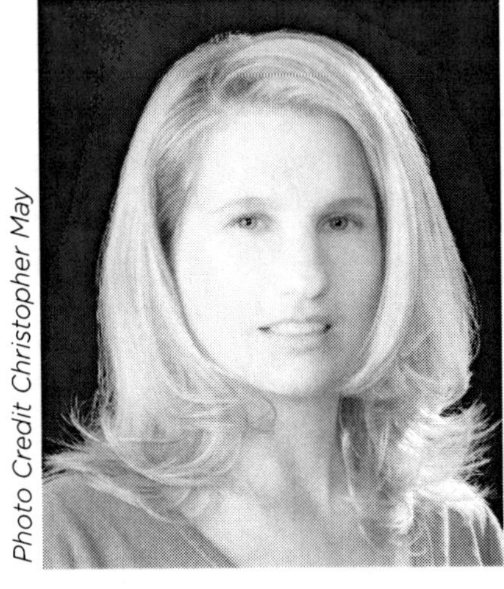

Photo Credit Christopher May

Deirdre Layne

Both healer and businesswoman, Deirdre Layne began her career as a practitioner of energy healing, having been extensively mentored by internationally acclaimed healers since 1989. After beginning her career in Los Angeles – where she was asked to participate in an NIH study on alternative medicine – she now maintains a healing practice in Atlanta, although the Earth Clinic communities are her primary focus.

As an outgrowth of that clinical practice, Ms. Layne founded EarthClinic.com, internationally recognized as one of the preeminent information providers on alternative medicine and healing. Deirdre is also a nationally ranked medalist in Traditional Karate, is a professional karate instructor, and holds a second-degree black belt. Deirdre earned her B.A. in Philosophy from Mount Holyoke College. She lives with her family in the Atlanta suburbs.

Daniel P. Kray

Ms. Layne chose author Daniel P. Kray to guide this book after working with him for several years on Earth Clinic sites. Deirdre selected him rather anonymously from a freelance contracting website. Yet his initial proposal so clearly stood out from among dozens in its vital energy, which exactly matched that of the Earth Clinic community, that the collaboration was a natural choice and has continued through several productive years and ventures.

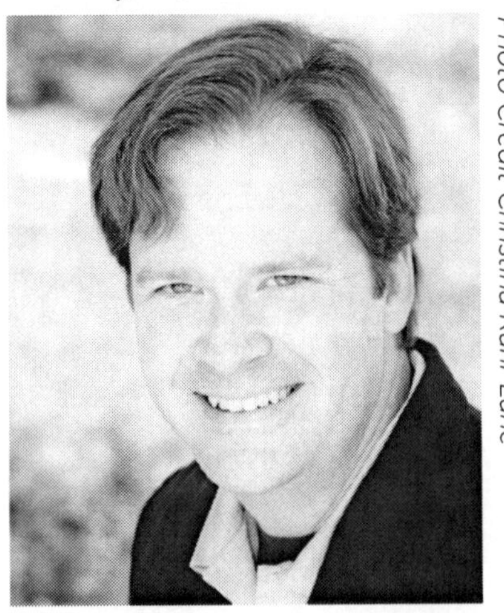

Photo Credit Christina Rahr Lane

For this project, Daniel calls on years of experience as a freelance writer and editor, previous work ghostwriting a memoir, and several years working as Senior Editor for Earth Clinic while taking part in that community. A graduate of Williams College with a B.A. in English and Philosophy, Mr. Kray has been Senior Writer and Editor for several websites in addition to magazine and other original work. His experience in publishing, education, travel (six continents), and knowledge of biology, medicine, and exercise prepared him for the Body Axis project. He is a resident of a bucolic New York village.

CPSIA information can be obtained at www.ICGtesting.com
Printed in the USA
LVOW07s1629270815

451782LV00034B/558/P